MW00478341

Summer's Complaint

*My family's courageous, century-long struggle
with a rare genetic cancer syndrome*

by Laura Kieger

This book is available for educational use. For information or to request discounted bulk quantities contact Critical Eye Publishing at 612.440.7107.

Summer's Complaint is a work of nonfiction. The stories and events are true and the people are real. Some names and identifying details have been changed to protect the privacy of individuals.

This book is not intended to be a substitute for the medical advice of a licensed physician. The reader should consult with their doctor in any matters relating to his/her health.

Internet references contained in this work are current at publication time, but Critical Eye Publishing cannot guarantee that a specific reference will continue to be maintained in any respect.

Edited by D.J. Schuette at www.criticaleyeediting.com
Cover Photography courtesy of North Dakota Tourism
Cover Design by Gabriel Vespasiano and D.J. Schuette
Rear cover DNA image courtesy of NIH.gov

First print edition, 2017
Printed in the United States of America.

ISBN: 978-0-9984293-3-5

Excerpt from "Kindness" from Words Under the Words: Selected Poems by Naomi Shihab Nye, copyright © 1995. Reprinted with the permission of Far Corner Books.

Critical Eye Publishing
Andover, Minnesota 55304

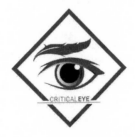

For my family, whose unwavering support made this book possible.
You are the most courageous people I have ever known.

Qu'Hier Que Demain

INTRODUCTION

He wore a cornflower blue satin suit. The same beautiful shade of his ever-curious eyes and the cherished threadbare baby blanket he'd once stroked while sucking his thumb. I had to stand on my tiptoes to see his face. He looked like he was sleeping, and I thought about those late afternoons that I'd snuck into his room waiting for him to wake from his nap so we could sing *Itsy Bitsy Spider* together. We'd laugh, my nephew and I, making a big circle with our arms over our heads when "out came the sun and dried up all the rain," and the itsy bitsy spider would climb up the spout again.

I'd never seen a dead person before. I wasn't sure how to act, so I took my cues from the adults around me. The grownups shuffled past Markie's tiny casket and conveyed their sympathies to my family. "So young," they said with a sad shake of their heads. "Such a shame." Or, "At least he isn't suffering any longer."

I watched my sister Karen's face. She had the same blue eyes as her son, the same fair skin and gentle nature. She looked tired as she warmly grasped outstretched hands—hands offered as a way to comfort the twenty-year-old mother of two who would have to do the unthinkable: bury her nearly three-year-old son. Mostly, I worried that our younger sister Lisa would start twirling around in her dress like a typical eight-year-old who has no idea how to behave in a funeral home. But I also wondered what I should say if anyone asked how I was feeling, or how my family was doing. All I could come up with for an answer was *"I don't know,"* because I hadn't even known that my nephew was dying—my parents hadn't told me. I was terrified that well-intentioned neighbors would take my hand and say, "We're so sorry," because I wasn't sure if I should smile and say, "Thank you," or gaze down at my shoes to hide what I was really feeling. And I couldn't turn to Lisa for help. She didn't understand the finality of death. Being a little kid has its advantages.

It was August 9, 1969. A Saturday. I woke and ambled sleepily into the kitchen. The smell of my father's freshly made Swedish egg coffee wafted through the room. Karen and Mom stood in front of the sink, talking quietly. I didn't think they saw me standing there in the doorway, but they stopped talking and their eyes locked. I sensed it was a serious, grownup conversation. Even at the age of ten, I knew that whatever they were discussing I wasn't prepared for it. But instead of running away, I looked down at the hem of my nightgown and waited for the bad news I knew must be coming.

"Markie died, Laura," my mom said. Then she and my sister turned back to the sink and continued talking in those hushed tones.

It was one of those moments where you find yourself dragged, unwillingly and ruthlessly, into adulthood. I'd just finished fourth grade and wasn't even interested in boys yet. I was hardly ready to come to terms with death. Much less the death of a small boy whose shoes I'd helped put on before we went out to play in the sandbox together and who'd spent countless hours snuggled on my lap as I read him his favorite stories. I stood there motionless trying to form some words—any words.

"You didn't tell me he was going to *die*," I said, spitting out the words with a vehement snarl. *"Why didn't you tell me?"*

The neckline of my nightgown was wet with tears, and I pulled it up in an attempt to cover my face. I felt betrayed. And hurt that none of them had seen me as adult enough or emotionally strong enough to be told the truth: that my nephew's chances of surviving the hepatoblastoma—a hard tumor cancer of his liver—were practically zero. Not even Mayo Clinic could save him. But the adults in my life hadn't prepared me for the inevitable. I was angry and suddenly much older than my ten-year-old self could process.

Less than a month before, I'd worn that same shade of blue as a junior bridesmaid in my sister Debbie's wedding. I had my hair done at a salon and wore white gloves and carried a basket of flowers. It was a stifling July day and the air conditioning was broken in the church, so I was glad to have my hair pulled up into a bun. I felt so special and almost grown up—not quite old enough to be a bridesmaid, but beyond the age of a flower girl.

All of Debbie's younger sisters and brothers were in the wedding—Karen, Butch, Marcie, Walt, me, Lisa, and Eric. My role, of course, was to make sure Lisa (a flower girl) and Eric (the ring bearer and youngest of the eight kids) stood where they were supposed to and played their part. I imagine it must have been hard on my parents to put on a brave face at the wedding knowing their grandson was terminally ill, and much more so for Karen. But as I got older, I realized that's the way my family is. We just don't fall apart. It must be the stoic Danish side in us, I guess.

So there I was, standing in the kitchen doorway with tears spilling down my cheeks, having just been told that Markie was dead. My junior bridesmaid dress was still draped over a chair in my bedroom instead of hanging neatly in the closet, as my mother had demanded. I felt sick. Sick knowing I'd been just a clueless kid all along and that the adults in my life hadn't told me he was going to die, or shared with me (as I found out later) that the doctors had given him "maybe six months."

Not long after his second birthday, Markie's dad had tossed him into the air and, upon catching him, felt a hard lump the size of an egg on the upper right side of his stomach. We all watched over the next few months as his abdomen swelled and his skin turned a sickly shade of yellow from jaundice. His arms and legs, instead of growing more muscled, became stick-thin, and his baby soft cheeks seemed to sink into his skull. Despite what was right in front of me, I'd fallen into that little kid magical thinking, assuming everything would turn out okay just because it *had to*. The doctors would have a plan to fix my nephew, because a happy and loved little boy doesn't get *that kind of sick*, and it's totally incomprehensible to a ten-year-old that he might actually *die*. And what about Jesus? I'd put in my time at Sunday school. Why couldn't He step in to stop a disease that strikes "one in a million?"

And besides, Auntie Del was the one who was *supposed* to die. I knew that because Mom had brought her Aunt Adele home to stay with Lisa and me in our bedroom so we could help take care of her. Adele wasn't related by blood, but through a previously annulled marriage to my mom's Uncle William. My mother always wanted us to call her Grandma Baker, but it never stuck. I would take Auntie Del's arm to steady her when she needed to stand to go to the bathroom. I'd bring a bowl to hold under her chin when she was feeling sick to her stomach. I brought her Kleenex and extra blankets when she needed them. We all knew *she* was dying—the Aunt who'd raised my mom and who had saved our family so many times we'd quit counting. She was well into her seventies with an advancing breast cancer. She didn't say much, but when she did she often prayed for God to take her and "not the baby." Maybe that was something I should have paid more attention to.

I vaguely recall what it was like being little—happy, carefree, and prone to magical thinking. But that time didn't last long, at least not as I remember it now.

It was 1963. The day before my fifth birthday I was sitting in front of the TV with Betsy McCall paper dolls and dresses lying in neat piles next to me on the rug. It was two weeks after President Kennedy had been assassinated. My mother was pregnant with Eric but didn't know it yet. On the afternoon news, I watched as my father—covered with a dark gray blanket and strapped to a stretcher—was carried up a ladder from a debris-filled hole. He'd been blown out of that hole and crashed back into it when a welding torch got too close to a propane tank at his job site. Auntie Del sobbed in the background.

Oblivious, I asked her if she had more magazines I could cut paper dolls from as she reached for the Kleenex.

My father's heart stopped on the way to the emergency room, and Pastor Grant from Faith Lutheran waited for my parents at the hospital, fully prepared to administer last rites. Miraculously, Dad made it through those first crucial hours, and by the end of his first week in the hospital, his condition had improved from critical to stable. But even during those days of intense worry and turmoil, I never had a sense of impending disaster all grown up and serious, no cloud of doom bearing down on my family.

Money was tight while my dad spent the better part of a year on our pull-out couch recovering from his injuries. Auntie Del paid our mortgage so we wouldn't lose the house. Our neighbors, the Curtises, bought our Christmas tree that year and dragged it over for us. I was thrilled, of course, having been cheated out of a decent birthday present due to the accident. My sister Marcie recounted years later the feeling of having to take a donated tree and a few gifts for the younger kids to open on Christmas day. She said she "hated being poor." But I never really felt the embarrassment of having to depend on the kindness of others like my older siblings did.

I shifted my gaze to the charm bracelet on my wrist. There were only two charms on it—one given to me by Debbie as a gift for being a part of her wedding party, the other a tiny round picture frame that held a photo of Markie on his first birthday. I twirled the bracelet around my wrist to keep my eyes on something other than Pastor Grant as he approached the small altar at the front of the room. I listened to the words of spiritual guidance that drifted over those who had gathered. I should have found those words comforting, but I didn't. If anything, they added to my confusion.

As mourners paid their respects and said their goodbyes to my nephew that August evening, I sensed a change within. A burgeoning maturity, certainly, and perhaps also a mistrust in the fairness of the universe that I was too young to define as cynicism. As the funeral director closed the lid of Markie's casket later that night, I swallowed a painful lump in my throat, and tears spilled down my cheeks. The finality of that moment was my first real taste of grief and marked the end of my childhood. The days of magical thinking were over.

What we didn't know in 1969 was why that small, loving child barely out of toddlerhood had developed an exceptionally rare liver cancer. Was it the "will" of some mean-spirited God? Or some terrible, freakish act of nature that just happened to befall our family? As it happened, it was merely the beginning of what we didn't know.

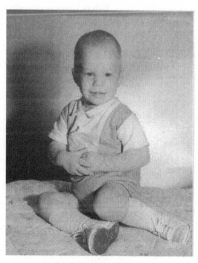

Markie, age 1

PART ONE:

Young Storyteller

CHAPTER 1: IMAGES AND WORDS

I always looked forward to watching the 8-millimeter films—also known as the "family movies." We'd excitedly go down to the basement to retrieve folding chairs in anticipation of a Friday or Saturday night filled with constant laughter and poking fun at one another while we watched. Mom would make popcorn as my dad made sure he could find the screen and tested the reels and bulb in the projector. Nothing extinguished our fun more than hearing him shout, "the light bulb is out!"

Over the years we became so familiar with what we were viewing we could often anticipate it. The Christmas stockings always hung above the fireplace in the same direction, starting with Debbie's on the far right and working their way over to Eric's on the left. Debbie and Karen in matching dresses, one of them in Mom's arms and the other in Dad's. My brother Jim or "Butch" (a name bestowed on him by the nurses when he was born) with a toy gun in hand, running around in a little bolero hat and bolo tie pretending to be Roy Rogers. Marcie, always with a bandage on one knee just visible under the hem of her dress and constantly looking anywhere other than at the camera; even in still photos, something else always seemed to capture Marcie's attention. Karen, in a bright white nurse's costume—complete with cape and hat—that she loved to dress up in. And Walt, standing by the doghouse in the backyard, thoughtfully watching over our dog Lassie and her puppies.

The only time I show up in the 8-millimeter films (by then in color) is an extended camera shot of me as a toddler in a holiday dress, clinging to our terrified cat. I look to be about two years old. My round face stands out and serves as a reminder to all where Debbie's "Pumpkin" nickname for me came from. I'm grinning and waving for the camera, sitting on a rug surrounded by stuffed animals beneath the Christmas stockings. Mine is the last on the left of the mantel signifying that I'm the youngest—a coveted position. I'd practically leap from my chair in sheer astonishment as I watched that rare footage where I was the center of attention for the next minute or two, at least on film. It was incontrovertible Kodachrome evidence that I was the youngest, most-adored child at that moment.

Other than that cherished shot, Lisa, Eric, and I rarely made an appearance in those 8-millimeter movies. We used to laugh that if it weren't for Grandma Evelyn's penchant for photography, the only pictures of us would have been those always-horrible school portraits that we all refused to give out to our classmates and friends. There were pictures of Lisa and Eric as infants—especially Eric, but no pictures exist of my first six months of life. It may not have always been that way...

My older brother Walt decided to pop popcorn in my parents' closet sometime in the early '60s. I would have been four or five at the time. There's a good chance I heard him in there, or at least had some inkling of what he was up to. I don't know exactly what happened, only that it involved a lack of supervision, a poorly thought out plan, matches, and a saucepan he'd taken from the kitchen. But after a while, even a little kid comes to understand that young boys in the presence of matches rarely ends well—be it in a closet popping popcorn, or smoking cigarettes in the attic above the garage.

After the fire department came and put the fire out, we discovered that many of the treasured photographs—so carefully stored in plastic boxes in that closet—had either been destroyed or damaged. We used to joke about the remaining photos, their edges singed and brown, as having "survived Walt's first ill-advised attempt at making popcorn." Thankfully, the 8-millimeters were stored in the linen closet in the hallway outside of our bedrooms, so those memories were spared. And even though Eric, Lisa, and I were bit players in the family movies, we still loved watching the films to see the younger parents our older siblings experienced. Our own experiences were much different. It was almost like watching another family.

My parents always looked so young and attractive in the films. I saw my dad as the "original Renaissance man," because he both played football and was in the drama club—a rare combination of thespian and athlete. My sister Debbie told me the girls in her kindergarten class used to swoon when my dad came to pick her up from school; he was so handsome and possessed one of those genuine, light-up-your-heart grins. My mom was an auburn-haired, green-eyed beauty who wore elegant strapless dresses to birthday celebrations and baptisms in the years before I was born. Yet in other films, we'd see her sans lipstick and in pants complete with a tied-at-the-waist flannel shirt when she and my dad went camping and fishing. This supported her claims of being a tomboy who rode horses and picked sleeping bats off the rafters in the barn during summer visits to Devils Lake when she was a fourteen-year-old heartbreaker.

Because my father's parents (my grandmother Evelyn and grandfather Walter) lived nearby (as opposed to my mother's side living in North Dakota), it was always easier to refer to the "Danish side" or the "Swedish side" when engaged in conversations regarding my extended family. I'd heard from my dad that his step-grandmother Anna, a Swedish immigrant, had once driven a horse-drawn carriage to Arizona in an effort to save her first husband from tuberculosis—the belief being that the warm, dry weather there might help him. Unfortunately, he passed away, and after a proper mourning period Anna remarried. She adopted Evelyn in the process, and moved her new family to Cambridge, Minnesota. As kids, we used to call Evelyn "little Grandma" and Anna "big Grandma"— whether because Anna was taller or older than Evelyn, I don't know. I never asked, but it seemed the accepted way for us to differentiate between the grandmas.

My grandfather Walter was a Danish immigrant from a family of seven kids. His uncle sponsored his trip to the United States and made sure he learned English and prepared himself for a job. He became a bricklayer, and he and Evelyn married and raised three boys, one of whom was my father, James Gerald or "Jerry." Walter never returned to Denmark despite desperate letters from his sister pleading for him to come home so they could meet his family and so he could see his parents again before they died.

By all accounts, my dad grew up in an energetic, testosterone-fueled home, which would not have been

Grandma Evelyn's preference. My grandfather, dad, and uncles Ron and Ken loved horsing around and played countless practical jokes on each other, while my grandmother steered clear of their nonsense. The daughters she'd always wanted finally came in the form of in-laws in the late 1940s when my dad and uncle married their sweethearts. My parents married in 1947 when they were both seventeen and still in high school. They even attended my dad's football team banquet as "Mr. and Mrs. Christensen."

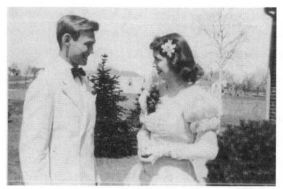

Prom Night, 1947

They lived in Walter and Evelyn's three bedroom, one bathroom brick Tudor in St. Paul. Soon enough, my parents brought four children into the fold, all born about a year apart: Deborah (1948), Karen (1949), James Gerald Jr. or "Butch" (1950), and Marcie (1952). In my grandmother's words, "they just kept coming."

I loved going to my grandparents' house growing up. Sundays were reserved for family time, and we'd have dinner there with my grandparents, uncles, aunts, and cousins almost every week. My grandfather raised roses, and I can still remember stopping at each and every one of the pink, red, or white rosebushes and sticking my pudgy face into them and inhaling their wonderful fragrance—I associated that smell with all the good things that had happened in that house. I learned how to whistle sitting on my great-grandmother's lap one afternoon after being deemed too young to go with the other kids to Como Zoo. She'd sing to us in Swedish and let us play with the dolls in her bedroom in the attic. In the summer, if we were really lucky, my grandfather would make us real malts using an old stainless steel malt mixer. Then we kids would fight over who'd be the lucky recipient of the last of the malted milk at the bottom of the mixer cup. And Grandma Evelyn always kept Fanny Farmer candy bars in her kitchen cupboard—that was the good chocolate. Everything about that house made me feel loved.

What the 8-millimeter films didn't show—and the black and white photos only gave a ghostly glimpse into—was the brief life of my mother's mother. My grandmother Cecilia died at age thirty-two when my mom was just six years old. My mother, Colleen, was her only child. Cecilia, however, had been the youngest of five siblings—William, Kathleen, Mayme, and Joseph preceded her. They were born to Henry and Mary Regan Baker and lived on a farm in Devils Lake. My mother spent summers at the family farm but lived with her Uncle William and Aunt Adele the rest of the year while attending an all-girls Catholic boarding school in Minnesota. Uncle William was an Army personnel officer, and Adele was a private duty nurse.

Grandma Cecilia had dark hair. I couldn't tell what color her eyes were, as all of the pictures of her were grainy black-and-whites or re-touched photos where someone had added a splash of pink to her cheeks. She kept her hair in a bob, fashionable for the time, and wore long pearl necklaces and sleeveless, fringed flapper-style dresses, which were also popular in the 1920s. According to her older sister Kathleen, they once went into town in Devils Lake after getting "gussied up" and had a photo taken at Slorby Studio, which years later made it into the local newspaper, captioned: "The Fabulous Baker Girls."

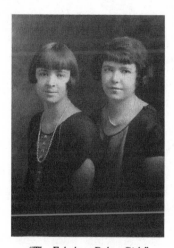

"The Fabulous Baker Girls"

The remaining pictures of Cecilia show her with my mom, her husband, Reginald, or as part of group shots where it's difficult to identify her. If not for Kathleen or Adele's handwriting on the back of the photos, I would have had trouble spotting her.

When I later asked my mother about her lineage, she mentioned only that they were Irish and Catholic, and that there may have been some horse thieves in the bunch. Even Guy Fawkes, the famous anarchist who was part of a group of conspirators who'd tried to blow up the British Parliament was allegedly on a branch of our family tree. Beyond that, she didn't easily share her recollections about family and her childhood.

My mom did once tell me, however, that the one thing she remembered about Grandma Cecilia's funeral was the overpowering smell of lilies. She forever hated that smell and used to say that when she died, there were to be no lilies at her own funeral.

One thing that is obvious from the pictures of my mother as a girl is that she loved animals. In many of them she's riding horses, taking her dog for a walk, or cuddling kittens. I know how much she enjoyed visits to the Connor farm and hanging out with her cousins Clinton, Erin, Donnie, and Mike. She and Erin were especially close, probably because they were the only girls.

Over time, I began to realize that what made my parents early years together seem so romantic and privileged were the people who made regular appearances in the old black and white photos and family movies. There was the almost constant presence of my grandparents, who took them in and provided a home for them and my older siblings until they were ready to establish a home of their own. My mom's Uncle William, Aunt Adele, Aunt Kathleen and Uncle Joe Connor provided my mother's familial thread back to Devils Lake. Close friends from Faith Lutheran Church in St. Paul. My uncles Ron and Ken and their wives, Grace and Carol. They all helped each other and looked out for one another. They were godparents to nieces and nephews and friends' children. It was the combination of an intergenerational home environment and a family devoted to one another and their Lutheran church that made it so special.

By the time my brother Walt came along in 1955, my parents had finally moved out of my grandparents' house and into their own home on Shryer Avenue in Roseville, complete with a big yard, a dog, a cat, and a couple of lambs. They'd settled in a neighborhood unlike a lot of the cookie-cutter neighborhoods that dotted the American landscape following the end of World War II. While there was criticism of the often dull housing developments everywhere else, my dad, his brothers, and my grandfather built my parents' first home on a double lot. The house was a brick three bedroom, one bath rambler with a full basement and single car garage. I never worried about the Big Bad Wolf or a Midwestern tornado destroying our home on Shryer. I felt safe there. Nothing would bring down the house the men in my family built.

CHAPTER 2: **HIGHCHAIRS AND HIJINKS**

I've always been suspicious of people who recall, sometimes in great detail and in vivid language, when they were born or when they took their first step. I, however, remember the first time I was aware that I was an individual separate from all the chaos that surrounded me. My first independent memory as a child found me seated in a highchair wearing a crinkly, itchy dress. I was presumably in the highchair because there was no chair for me at the kitchen table, and my sister Lisa, the new youngest, would have been in my mom's lap. There were lots of people in the house, and I can remember a tall blonde man with a deep booming voice that I later attached to my dad's friend, Fred. I was wedged into a tight corner between the refrigerator and the kitchen wall so that I was out of the way. The fact that I was trapped in the highchair just made my aggravation worse. A small plate of food and a plastic glass of milk sat on the tray in front of me, but they didn't stay there for long. I remember it in slow motion (which makes it seem even more calculated)—I dumped the milk on the floor and pushed the plate off the tray. My little tantrum taught them an important lesson: don't push a toddler who'd recently lost her special youngest child status out of the way.

Lassie and the cat happily helped clean up my mess.

I don't remember Lisa's birth in 1961. She and I were too close in age. One day I just lost my coveted place as the youngest. I'd hung on to it for two and a half years, and then she showed up due to my parents' apparent inability to keep their hands off of each other.

The most vivid memory I have of Lisa as a small child— other than her following me around constantly—was her penchant for running away. I'd be just home from kindergarten trying to eat my chicken noodle soup in peace, and my mom would suddenly notice Lisa wasn't playing in the sandbox anymore. All hell would break loose, I'd be recruited to help track her down, and my soup would sit forgotten and cold on the table. The usual suspect was a boy about Lisa's age named Ralphie who lived behind us on Skillman Street. When Lisa went missing, Ralphie would often be her accomplice. On several occasions, they'd find one another and decide to go exploring. More than once, their adventures involved the Roseville Police Department. In one memorable incident, they'd toddled about four blocks along a busy road and were found very close to State Highway 36. It's a wonder they weren't killed.

Fortunately, Ralphie eventually moved out of the neighborhood, and Lisa, thankfully, grew out of her wandering stage.

I do remember Eric being born, because it was the August after my dad was blown out of his boots in the work site explosion that nearly killed him. Kid number eight arrived on August 25, 1964, while my dad more or less lived on our couch with a cast on his leg from foot to hip. But I wasn't annoyed by Eric's arrival like I'd been by Lisa's. Instead, I found him enchanting. He was beautiful. Dark blue eyes and a perfect face. I was only allowed to hold him while sitting down, as he came into the world tipping ten pounds. I'd watch him through the slats in his crib, waiting for him to wake up, much like I later would with Markie.

Eric was a strong Scandinavian name. His middle name, Howard, came from my mom's war hero uncle—a Darby Ranger killed in World War II after parachuting behind enemy lines as part of a demolition team. Despite Eric being the eighth child in our family (a classmate's entry in Debbie's yearbook read, "I can't believe your mom had another baby!"), and though he came along during a challenging financial time, we all adored him. Eric certainly didn't feel like a burden. In fact, we couldn't get enough of him. Lisa and I thought him so beautiful, we once dressed him in one of Lisa's old rompers and a bonnet and pushed him around the driveway in his stroller. He looked just like we had as babies, blonde curls and all. My dad pulled up after work, and when he saw what we were doing, he quickly picked Eric up, plopped him in the front seat of the truck, and drove him to the nearest barbershop. When Eric returned, his lovely blonde curls were gone.

Curls or no curls, Eric as a tiny boy was endlessly energetic. He was once traumatized by one of the big male gorillas at Como Zoo. It must have stuck its tongue out at him (or something similarly sinister) and at two years old, Eric didn't respond particularly well. He became utterly paranoid that gorillas were on their way to our house to devour us and leave a big, smelly mess in their wake.

On another memorable occasion, Eric somehow pried his way into a bottle of what my parents called "pep pills." My mom took them occasionally when she needed to stay awake to take care of us during the day after working a night shift at the Rose of Sharon nursing home. She didn't work those shifts often, but did so occasionally to make extra money. Before the open pill bottle was discovered on the kitchen counter around 3:00 a.m., Eric was up and running around the house like a pint-sized maniac. He jumped around in front of my bedroom window while pointing up at the Wallraffs' house, absolutely convinced that gorillas were lumbering down their driveway. Somehow, Lisa slept through the ruckus. I initially found it amusing, but when he wouldn't stop chattering and dashing from room to room, I realized there was something wrong with him. The hallway light came on before I could wake my parents; they were already up, alerted by the noise. The evidence in the kitchen told the story. At the ER, the doctors pumped his stomach of the offending pep pills, but not even they could resolve Eric's gorilla phobia. Exasperated with all of it, my mom came up with a clever idea. She gave Eric a bunch of cloves and told him to sprinkle them around the perimeter of our entire yard, both front and back. She told him that gorillas hate cloves—it was supposedly the equivalent of a vampire's aversion to garlic. It took him days to finish, but he did it all by himself.

And Mom was right, too. We never had a gorilla come to our house.

When I was bit older than four, it wasn't unlike me to be asking my parents and siblings a constant string of questions and demanding they read me anything I could get my hands on. We read the Sunday comics and National Geographic magazines together. We also had a set of encyclopedias purchased using gold bond stamps from the Red Owl grocery store that my mom licked and stuck into a savings book. I'd pull one of the encyclopedia volumes off of the bookshelf and toss it to whoever was sitting on the couch in our living room, crawl onto their lap and demand immediate reading attention. To counteract this despairing dependency on others, I was determined to learn to read as quickly as I could. At some point, my mom bought me my very own Dr. Seuss beginner books. She read them to me, and when I mastered sounding out the words, I read them to Lisa while restraining her so she couldn't escape. I couldn't get enough of this newly acquired skill and practiced reading everything from the back of cereal boxes to my older siblings' report cards. The great downside to all of this was that I'd sometimes get my active hands on things not meant for my eyes: papers that had survived the Great Popcorn Fire of 1962 in the plastic boxes in my parents' bedroom closet, notes, cards, legal records, letters from relatives (some of whom I'd never met). The important documents were stuffed in a large silver box with a lock that was seldom used. They also had a green, army-type metal box under their bed that they did keep locked, but other than that, nothing in the house was safe from my insatiable curiosity.

My first grade teacher's name was Mrs. Collins. She saw something in me from the very beginning of the school year. She placed me in the "high" reading group, my precocious insistence to learn to read paying off. Mrs. Collins trusted me to be class monitor when she had to step out of the room. She encouraged my writing. I remember feeling special despite being but one of thirty kids in my class, whereas at home I felt like one of eight constantly vying for attention. My favorite book was *Mr. Popper's Penguins*, which fueled a short-lived obsession with the flightless birds that spilled over into my poems and drawings. I wore a favorite dress every day I could get away with it until winter came; it had a checked pattern in fall colors with small leaves embroidered on a white collar. It was a dress of my very own and not one of the usual hand-me-downs. Auntie Del had bought it for me before I started school that year. She'd been the one to take me school shopping for clothes and shoes and took me to see the dentist. As always, we ended our busy day of shopping at Sears in a booth in the department store's cafe sharing a tulip sundae.

While grade school provided some much-needed structure for my childhood days, my home environment was frequently in stark contrast. There was always an element of risk, especially when my parents would leave us home with the babysitter—otherwise known as our sister Marcie. A sure sign they were going out without us was the appearance of chicken pot pies or Swanson fried chicken TV dinners in the oven on a Friday or Saturday night. The mayhem started shortly after supper.

We had a laundry chute in the bathroom closet where we could drop dirty clothes onto the basement floor below, right in front of the washing machine. I loved to shove things down that laundry chute. Smelly cloth diapers. Stuffed animals. My sister Lisa. I didn't want to hurt her or anything, so I always made a big pile of dirty clothes—smelly diapers included—as a crash pad for her. I knew she'd fit because she was small and skinny. Just to be sure, I suggested she keep her arms firmly at her sides during her trip. After all, I'd be on the receiving end of a good spanking if there were any obvious signs of physical trauma on Lisa when my parents returned. Luckily for me, she dropped through that fifteen-inch square opening in the bathroom floor like a little human missile and landed safely below. What started out as a potentially dangerous homemade thrill ride ended with her pounding back up the stairs exclaiming, "Let's do it again!" Eric kept his distance, watching our antics from the safety of his toddler trike, one hand on the handlebars and the other clutching a well-gummed Gerber cookie, unaware that he was only a year or two away from his first laundry chute launching.

Another example of a risky though rewarding event on those evenings of nominal supervision was the roasting of marshmallows in our fireplace. I was in charge of gathering the sticks. Lisa would climb up on the kitchen counter in search of marshmallows. Marcie would track down the matches and start a fire. We were careful to always open the flue, otherwise the house would fill with smoke, potentially bringing our fun to an abrupt end. We never had the patience to roast them to a golden brown, so the goal was to have your marshmallows ignite like flaming napalm. It was a thing of beauty. No one ever got burned, but plenty of those singed, gooey firebombs landed on the carpet. We'd spend hours trying to scrub the burn marks out with Brillo pads, but our attempts were mostly futile. Amazingly, my parents never mentioned them. I think they were just happy for the opportunity to sneak out of the house without kids once in a while.

After Eric, Lisa, and I miraculously survived our early childhoods, we eventually became full-fledged members of an especially large gaggle of kids lovingly known as the "Neighborhood." Debbie, Karen, Butch, Marcie and Walt had all been part of the Neighborhood as well, but they were well into their pre-teen and teenage years by the time we were allowed to roam about untethered and unsupervised. It was a bit like being set free. And we took full advantage of that newfound freedom.

CHAPTER 3: THE NEIGHBORHOOD

When I remember the neighborhood in which I grew up, it's always as an amusing and inseparable combination of both people and place. Along with our family of eight kids, collectively referred to as "The Christensens," there were the Wallraffs' seven kids, and the Wilsons' nine kids. Our three families alone could singlehandedly perform minor miracles— like coordinating a baseball game or a round of Midnight Ghostlight after dark in the summer—due to our sheer numbers. Then there were the Hinrichs, the Schultzes, the Deutches, the Curleys, the Dunns, the Markgrafs, and the Bostons who lived on the street behind us that rounded out our neighborhood's contribution to the American Dream.

In terms of place, the neighborhood was extraordinary. I don't think our parents planned it that way, it just happened. It wasn't so much about keeping up with the Joneses or the nearby shopping malls and libraries as much as it was the natural habitat surrounding our street. We had access to massive amounts of open space. More than one hundred acres of woods and field to run and play in were right outside of our front doors. To the south we had the St. Paul Water Works, home to a thirty million gallon underground water reservoir operated by the City of St. Paul. It was hilly terrain with lots of pine trees, wetlands, prairie grass, and savanna. Best of all, there were no adults anywhere around—well, except for maybe one. Back in the sixties and seventies, a guy we all referred to as the "dean" supposedly guarded the Reservoir and surrounding woods. He allegedly possessed a pepper gun and wasn't afraid to use it. No one knew where this dean lived, but I'd always assumed it was the big white house just on the edge of the Reservoir. Every now and then, my brother Walt and his friend Dave would run up to me and my friends while we were building a fort in the woods yelling, "The dean is coming! The dean is coming!" Of course, we were terrified and would scatter like cockroaches startled by a sudden light. Frankly, I think the "dean" was just a made-up madman—an urban legend created to keep the kids out of there that passed from one generation to the next. To my knowledge, no one ever actually saw this mysterious person. The Reservoir was a place we could hide out in all day—building forts, picking asparagus, pretending we were characters in a Grimm's Fairy Tale. And if it rained, we could hide in one of the giant, empty water pipes that were stored near the Reservoir; four or five of us could easily crawl into one of those dark, claustrophobia-inducing metal monsters.

To the west at the end of our street was the Wallraffs' property, famous for its gigantic sledding hill. The Wallraff house sat atop the hill, which allowed Mrs. Wallraff to keep a watchful eye on us as we tobogganed or sledded down their front yard, all the while honing our reflexes to narrowly avoid crashing into the big trees at the bottom. Behind the Wallraffs' property was a large field. It was basically open prairie and served as a pasture for horses owned by a local family who also tended Roselawn Cemetery. The horses would wander up to the Wallraffs' fence, and we'd feed them apples. I loved it, and we could time their arrival to greet us at the fence to the hour. There was one black gelding named Nehru that seemed to lead the herd. He'd rear his head and stomp his weathered hooves in front of the other horses. He was the only reason I didn't climb under the fence to try to get closer to them. I imagined owning my own horse someday, so whenever I was out in the field and came across an abandoned halter or feed bucket, I'd pick it up and put it into the "someday I'm going to own a horse" box that I kept in my bedroom closet.

North of the field was a pond. Not a particularly clean pond, mind you—the water was more like runoff—but we had access to a small warming house to hang out in during the winter, and we could walk down there to skate or play broomball when it froze over. In the summer, it was a great place to catch turtles or jump into from a rope swing to cool off—if you didn't mind a little sludge.

On top of all that, the empty lot between two houses on the south side of my street served as a softball field. An almost-real softball diamond, not just a puny Wiffle ball diamond like the ones we carved out in our front yard. We'd spend hours every day each summer playing softball in that lot without ever having to worry about breaking a window or hitting a passing car, because the lot was at an incline, built into a small hill. We situated home plate below second base, so the balls we hit standing at home plate were either caught by an outfielder or rolled down the hill back to us, avoiding the street or any nearby windows. It was a masterpiece of natural engineering. I existed between all of these places—the Reservoir, the field behind the Wallraffs' house and the hill their house was situated on, the pond, and the empty lot. As the scorching summer sun dipped low in the sky, I'd listen for my mom's legendary two-finger whistle, calling me home for supper.

Life as a kid on Shryer Avenue in the late 1960s was never boring. My friends Kim, Linda, and I all had younger brothers the same age, which served us well. Whether we were putting on a play or a haunted house in the garage, we had a captive audience at our disposal. If we were playing pretend school, they were our pretend students whether they liked it or not. But at the same time, we defended our brothers fiercely and fearlessly. I remember Eric walking up our street one day with tears streaming down his face, saying that a "skinny blonde kid" had taken his bike down by the pond. I knew immediately it was that sneering, pimply-faced psychopath Paul who lived several blocks from our house. He was my age and taller than me, but he was scrawny—his chest was practically concave. He regularly picked on the younger kids. A real loser. I rounded up one of the Wallraff twins, and we raced down to the pond where Paul and three or four of his misfit buddies were standing on the shoreline pitching rocks into the water. Without a word, I charged him full bore and rammed my head into his gut, knocking him back into the water. He came up gasping and sputtering. While he tried to regain his composure, my super-girl sidekick retrieved Eric's bike from the pond, the handlebars peeking from the green, slime-skimmed water. As we walked away with it, I tossed a look over my shoulder and with a bit of bravado said, "And if you ever go near my brother again, I'll bring my big sister with me, and she'll really pound on you." The best part was the ribbing he endured from his friends later—"Paul got his ass kicked by a girl!" As bold as it seems, back then boys wouldn't dare hit a girl, so my aggressive tactic wasn't overly risky. Plus, replacing Eric's bike would have been an expense that my parents couldn't easily afford.

Surviving a typical Minnesota winter was every bit as challenging as combating neighborhood bullies. We had a wind chill chart on the side of our refrigerator next to a copy of the Serenity Prayer. It was frayed and hung from the refrigerator with tape, but it served its purpose. We'd take our index fingers, find the outside temperature on the left axis of the chart and then follow the grid on the chart by the forecast for the wind speed that day on the lower axis of the chart. Where they met would tell us the "true" temperature or "how it feels on exposed skin." I remember getting ready for school in the winter and checking the chart. If it was twenty-five below outside with an expected fifteen to twenty mile per hour wind, it warned that "exposed human flesh could freeze in less than ten minutes" and touted an "extreme risk of hypothermia." Once I saw that, I knew my mom would be pushing the full cover up: hats, mittens, and if she had her way, scarves covering our mouths and noses. I always hated wearing a hat, but Mom insisted we'd lose heat through our heads, so I never managed to escape the house without one. By the time I reached the end of the driveway, it was shoved deep into my coat pocket. The one thing that eased the fear of freezing flesh, however, was the knowledge that Mom would make chocolate pudding for breakfast on the stove. She'd serve it to us piping hot with whipped cream on the top, which began to melt the minute she dished it up in our bowls. That's right—chocolate pudding for breakfast. It made getting up and preparing to stand out at the bus stop on those bitterly cold mornings so much more bearable.

Apparently inspired by the scene in *The Sound of Music* where Julie Andrews pulls down the drapes to make play clothes for Captain Von Trapp's children, my mother found an inexpensive, heavy, blue-quilted material at Minnesota Fabrics and decided to sew us all winter jackets one year. While I coveted the plaid coats with cute fur collars and winter muffs I saw the other girls my age wearing, we got the boring jackets with industrial strength zippers. They looked like straight-up, Russian Army-issued winter parkas. My dad had her make one for him, and from there my mother furiously sewed one for Walt, Lisa, Eric, and me. Imagine us at the bus stop looking like recently released Gulag prisoners from Siberia. I remember walking into Lexington Elementary wearing that damn blue jacket and hanging it up on my coat hook while trying to avoid the eyes of the girl standing next to me. The fabric cost no more than fifty-five cents a yard. I silently cursed my mother for her humiliating thriftiness.

We'd occasionally bear witness to the practical joker in my dad when we were kids. One prank was especially horrific, while at the same time had me laughing so hard I had to lock myself in my bedroom afterward because my mom was not amused. As I recall it, my niece Shelby was visiting and about three years old. She had a terrible fear of clowns. There was a rubber clown mask sitting on the top shelf of my parents' bedroom closet, along with a hand buzzer. (The latter was an item I brought to school with me one day, a misguided idea that led to recess in an uncomfortable wooden chair in the principal's office.) Dad put on the clown mask and lay down on the living room couch with a pillow over his head.

"Shelby, come and help Grandpa. I can't breathe," he called.

I heard her running down the hallway. *I can't believe he's going to do this*, I thought, stifling giggles with a fist pressed to my mouth. Sure enough, she pulled the pillow off his face, and he sat straight up cackling menacingly. She tore out of the living room screaming for her grandmother like a banshee. One might expect this devious act to have left mental and emotional scars on my poor niece, but quite to the contrary, my mother again saved the day. She brought a sniveling and terrified Shelby back into the living room by the hand. As she consoled her, she explained that it was only Grandpa behind the mask and that all clowns were just people wearing a mask or face paint. Shelby recovered from her fear of clowns after that. The alternative would almost certainly have been years of therapy.

Along with my father's many handy talents—homegrown meteorologist, master gardener, current events watcher, and bricklayer extraordinaire—we could also count on him to follow speeding squad cars and fire engines. One eventful Sunday evening after family dinner at my grandparents', my dad spotted a fire engine with sirens blaring and lights blazing up ahead. I could see the grin spread across my dad's face in the station wagon's rearview mirror as he gunned the engine and fell in behind. The truck was a real beauty—a giant hook and ladder with at least eight firemen hanging off of it. We tailed it all the way down Larpenteur until it turned into our neighborhood. It sped down the hill toward our street when one of the firemen dangling from the side stuck his arm out to signal a left turn.

"Holy cripes," I exclaimed. "One of the neighbor's houses must be on fire!"

Mom and Dad didn't panic until we followed the engine onto our street and then watched the firemen point to the smoke billowing from our roof. My dad hadn't even slammed the station wagon into park before my mom burst out of the car screaming at the firefighter standing on our roof with an ax.

"It's just a turkey in the oven on a timer! The timer must have malfunctioned," she shouted hysterically.

It was chaos. The neighbors stood outside of their houses watching the battle of Colleen versus the firemen. We'd just bought a new oven, and she was sure that the timer feature was faulty. Fortunately, she was right. I was just glad the remaining pictures of us in my parents' bedroom closet were spared. I'd come to believe our family's often ill-fated relationship with fire might bring the Christensen house down after all. Between Walt's popcorn-popping experiment, the many evenings of roasting of marshmallows in the fireplace without adult supervision, and the faulty oven timer, I was convinced we'd eventually tempt fate one too many times. I just hoped I wouldn't be there when it happened.

CHAPTER 4: **WISE WORDS**

After Marcie left home in 1970 to start college at the University of Minnesota, I was the oldest of the sisters living in my parents' house. That was also the summer that I determined what I didn't want for *my* future.

I went inside to cool down after a scorching day of playing basketball in the Hinrichs' driveway. We didn't have air-conditioning, so all the windows were open but the shades were drawn to keep the house cool. I walked into the kitchen and opened the freezer—thankfully, there were still a couple of cherry popsicles left. I grabbed one and walked back toward our living room where my mom had been folding clothes with one of those big box fans blowing straight on her. The four youngest kids still living at home (Walt, me, Lisa, and Eric) coupled with my father's construction job generated a lot of laundry—piles of folded clothes sat on the couch. Mom was on the phone with someone from Como Zoo, asking how to become a foster parent to one or both of the new tiger cubs that had been making a big splash on the evening news.

A tiger cub living here? With us? I thought maybe she'd lost it.

I heard her say, "No, we don't have a fenced yard, but we could certainly install one if that's necessary."

What? I thought, incredulous. We'd spent the spring and summer of '65 chasing Lisa and Ralphie all over the neighborhood and *now* we'd invest in a fence? Was she serious? We had kids, dogs, cats, birds, hamsters, ducks, lambs, fish, and chameleons at any given time. Wasn't that enough? Couldn't she adopt a horse? Normally, I'd have been open to such an adventure, but I was changing. I blamed the summer heat for this obviously deranged idea of hers.

I knew my mom loved animals, but she had a semi-disabled husband whose worsening rheumatoid arthritis made just getting out of bed in the morning difficult, kids at home, and limited disposable income with which to take in a tiger or two, let alone feed them. I was entering sixth grade, and with Marcie going off to college, I was on the cusp of having my own room. I'd be damned if I was going to share it with Lisa or tiger cubs. I deserved my own space. I wanted the crazy to stop. It might be too late for my mother, but it wasn't for me. I would not marry young or become a young mother—that was tantamount to being handed your entire life's script at seventeen or eighteen years old.

While hiding in that hallway eavesdropping on my mother's phone conversation, I had mixed emotions. I might not have had everything that I wanted, but my parents had managed to provide the things that I needed. Yet I wanted more than they'd had. Moving out of the house and obtaining an education became my goal. I just needed to stay focused on my schoolwork and graduate with decent grades and an SAT score that would catch the eye of a college admissions officer.

That was my plan, and I made it that very moment while silently watching and listening to my mom on the phone.

Naturally, being the oldest girl in the house—which thankfully remained tiger-free—came with additional chores, but I never really minded "kitchen duty." Once I'd cleaned up after dinner and thrown some dishes in the dishwasher my Auntie Del had bought us years before, I could then sit down at the table and have coffee with whoever was at the table that night. Some of the most profound insights into my family's history came during those after-dinner conversations. Sometimes from my mom, and occasionally from my Great-Aunt Kathleen when she visited from Devils Lake, but the biggest revelations always came from Grandma Evelyn or "Gram" as we kids sometimes called her when we got older.

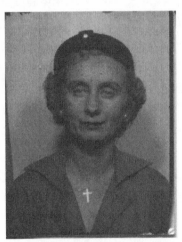

Grandma Evelyn (Gram), circa 1947

My conversations at that table with my grandmother were on a completely different level. After she was widowed in April of 1970, she'd drive over to our house every evening for dinner and after-dinner coffee complete with some sweet dessert Mom had made. Years later when we worried about her driving, one of us would go pick her up, bring her to our house, and then take her back to her apartment. And every evening is not an exaggeration—she made the trip through snowstorms and summer tornado watches for nearly twenty years. It didn't feel odd to me. It was just a continuation of what we'd done for many years when I was growing up—getting together as a family over a meal.

When Evelyn and I chatted, it was often just the two of us still sitting there after the table had been cleared. I remember well the conversations we'd have about my parents as a young married couple; I couldn't get enough of them. But the best part was that I always knew when she was being honest with me because of my covert childhood investigations into family documents. My grandmother had a knack for revealing family secrets in such a way that she wouldn't wind up in trouble with my dad. Between the two of us, we were particularly well-equipped to get to the bottom of things.

One kitchen table conversation we had in the early fall of 1970 surprised me and has stuck with me all these years. She recalled sitting at her own kitchen table back in 1947 right after my parents married at the age of seventeen, trying to get to know my mother a bit. I imagined the setting: my grandparents' kitchen had a small stainless steel table and chair set with red seat cushions that sat under a window looking out on my grandfather's rose bushes and their backyard. The yellow baker-man cookie jar sat on the counter, probably half full of sugar or gingerbread cookies just like it always was. It was the perfect setting for letting your guard down.

The young woman in front of her was suddenly thrust into the family, and a blind date, prom, and the subsequent quick elopement in Iowa hadn't given Evelyn much time to get to know her new daughter-in-law. Based on my recollection of that conversation with Gram, my impression was that it had been part friendly chat and part investigative interview designed to make sure she got "the good stuff."

Naturally, they talked about my mom's ancestry. Her mother, Cecilia, was Irish Catholic, her father, Reggie, Scotch and Protestant. When Cecilia died, she went to live with her Uncle William and his wife Adele. When my mom was fifteen, William left his wife and my mom, determined to obtain a divorce and an annulment and succeeded in both. Auntie Del was devastated. At this point in the conversation, my grandmother probably had a pretty good picture in her mind of my mother's childhood: a devoutly Catholic home environment, shuffled around a bit like most "military brats" due to her uncle's job with the Army, bouncing in and out of her biological father's life, caught in the middle of her guardian's unraveling marriage and then marrying young and not finishing high school. Not satisfied with what she'd learned to that point she asked more pointed questions about my mom's family.

"Well," my mother continued, "Auntie Kathleen is married to a man named Joe Connor. They have four kids of their own and also helped raise my Aunt Mayme's three kids after she died."

"And how old was Mayme when she died?" Grandma Evelyn asked. Thirty-two? And Cecilia died at age thirty-two? And what about your uncle Joseph? He died at thirty-nine? At this point, I can envision my grandmother sitting across that table from my mother, closing her eyes, and thinking very carefully about her next questions. "So in your mother's family, she and two of her siblings all died in their thirties? How?"

With a bit more prodding my grandmother learned that not long before they died, Joe, Mayme, and Cecilia all had something the family referred to as "summer's complaint." They got sick and died from whatever was ailing them.

I never quite understood how "summer" played into it. According to my mother, "summer's complaint" was more a reference to the symptoms, rather than the diagnosis, although the diagnoses all seemed suggestive of cancer—diarrhea, dramatic weight loss, lack of energy, and eventually death. It wasn't anything unusual to my mother, of course, because her grandmother, Mary Regan Baker, had died of the same thing. In fact, Mary's father, Peter Regan had brought her to Mayo Clinic in Rochester, Minnesota in 1911 to see if the doctors there could help her.

Gram told me that she'd once heard of something called "summer complaint," a childhood diagnosis given to unusual bouts of vomiting and diarrhea in infants and toddlers attributed to spoiled milk or fruit that had been left in the sun too long.

"But Mom always referred to it as summer's complaint. With an 's,'" I said.

"Maybe they'd once heard of summer complaint and adopted it for their symptoms, mistakenly adding the 's,'" she replied with a shrug. "You have to understand, I was very worried for your mother. I thought there might be something wrong with your mother's family."

She then explained that she'd spent the better part of a year sending letters, and obtaining death certificates from Bismarck, North Dakota.

"Your mom's Aunt Adele was particularly helpful," she told me. "She filled me in on many of the details that my inquiries couldn't answer."

"What did you do then?" I asked.

"Well Loll Doll," she said, using her nickname for me, "I did the only thing I could think of to do. I went to the library to do some research."

Evelyn had an unshakable fear that the untimely deaths of Mary, Joe, Mayme, and Cecilia were connected and caused by something that ran in my mom's family. Armed with a trove of medical information about my mom's relatives, Gram took the city bus down to the St. Paul City Library. She would have wandered the four floors, finally settling in the area that housed the non-fiction science and medical related books. She may have pulled some reference materials. She would have struggled to cobble together any published information that existed at that time for the general public on familial diseases. But she was determined to find out why three siblings from a single family from Devils Lake, North Dakota died in their thirties.

Sometime around 1956 or 1957, Evelyn noticed my mom had lost weight, hadn't been feeling well, and, as she put it, didn't look good. "I insisted she see a doctor because we were all very worried about her," she told me.

Her doctor determined she needed a thorough medical workup to include a family history and some specific diagnostic tests. Based on those findings, he recommended a consult with Dr. William Bernstein, a specialist in colorectal surgery and an early pioneer in the field of colon and rectal surgery at the University of Minnesota. What Dr. Bernstein found was a carpet of precancerous villous adenomatous polyps in my mother's colon—hardly the normal colon of an otherwise healthy female in her twenties. He would have seen this before in his practice, albeit rarely, and knew she needed immediate surgery to remove as much of her colon as possible to avoid a near inevitable—and potentially deadly—colorectal cancer.

The stress on my parents as they faced this surgery was immense. With five young children at home between the ages of nine and two (Debbie, Karen, Butch, Marcie and Walt), my mother and father had some serious decisions to make. Where should she have the surgery? Was Dr. Bernstein really the best surgeon in town? How would the kids be cared for while she recovered—*if* she recovered—because the surgery had major risks. And my mother's relatives had concerns, too. What if she didn't make it? Would she go to heaven or hell? Purgatory? She'd married a Lutheran and her children had been baptized in the Lutheran Church, but as far as we knew, she still considered herself Roman Catholic.

That Dr. Bernstein was Jewish was another concern. Mom's surgery was scheduled at Bethesda (a Lutheran Hospital) and not at St. Joseph's where her Uncle William would have preferred it take place. He thought it would be best to find a Catholic surgeon in a Catholic hospital with a Catholic priest standing by to perform last rites "just in case." My dad worried most about losing the love of his life and how he'd raise five kids on his own should the worst happen.

Luckily, Dad was the kind of person who could rise above the noise and focus on what was important. And as far as he was concerned, Uncle William's credibility as a model of moral virtue ended when he walked out on Adele, leaving her alone to raise my teenage mother.

As I listened to Gram tell the story, I found myself feeling just as sorry for my dad as my mom. The worry about potentially losing his young wife and mother of his children coupled with a family patriarch attempting to interfere in her medical care must have been extremely difficult for him.

In the end, the surgery was a success. Mom lost several feet of her colon, but she survived and regained her health. I was born a little over a year later.

CHAPTER 5: **SYNDROME**

It was September 1971, and the first day of seventh grade was around the corner. I was both excited and terrified. I'd somehow aced my clarinet audition for band and ended up placed in "first chair." Who would have guessed that practicing over the summer to alleviate boredom would improve my clarinet playing skills? I wanted to keep my winning streak going, so I asked my mom to sew me an outfit for my first day at Parkview Junior High. I'd recovered from the dreadful winter of homemade blue winter coats with my dignity still intact, so I was willing to give her another chance. I actually enjoyed picking out the pattern and material with her at Minnesota Fabrics. She convinced me to go with something splashy so I'd stand out among a sea of teenage girls wearing hip huggers and peasant blouses. We settled on a bright yellow polyester. The outfit included a vest with yellow ribbon that crisscrossed in the front and short shorts or "hot pants" as we called them back in those days. With money I'd earned babysitting, I also purchased a new pair of shoes—a combination light and dark brown saddle shoe with heels. And white knee-high socks. I was going for a cool Marcia Brady from *The Brady Bunch* look but ended up looking more like Jodi Foster's young prostitute character in the movie *Taxi Driver*. Not the wisest choice.

I knew within a few minutes of walking into Parkview Junior High that it wasn't a good look for me. In no way had I wanted to attract the attention of the older boys who stared at me as I fumbled with my locker, some of them with hints of moustaches above their lips. Deep voices and facial hair—good grief, how I missed grade school. Wandering the new hallways trying to figure out where my classes were, I felt small and vulnerable. I hated that feeling and couldn't wait to go back home and change my clothes. I never wore the outfit again.

In spite of my embarrassing first day of junior high, Parkview offered limitless possibilities. As in grade school, activities other than field trips were free and there were lots of extra-curricular activities we could join without worrying about fees or dues: co-ed dances, girls' sports like basketball, volleyball, and even synchronized swimming, drama club, and student council. Parkview had just recently opened, and it was considered state-of-the-art in the early seventies. It housed a pool and hockey rink, ball fields, and classrooms dedicated to wood shop, art, and home economics. And, it was in walking distance from our neighborhood.

Also within walking distance was a small ski resort called Villa, or "Mount Villa" as we sarcastically dubbed it. Some wise and wonderful people with the City of Roseville decided to turn a couple acres of hilly land into a local downhill ski destination. It was certainly nothing fancy—basically just two large hills separated by a towrope. The "chalet" was nothing more than a trailer that served up hot chocolate, apple cider, and a couple different kinds of candy bars. That was it. For kids my age, it was the place to be in wintertime. We couldn't get enough of that neighborhood marvel. Some of my friends didn't even ski; they just hung out in the chalet. There were no parents around either, just a guy, barely eighteen and smelling of marijuana, who took our money in exchange for lift tickets.

I quickly gave up any lingering notions of owning a horse and instead begged my parents to buy me a pair of nice skis, boots, and poles. They did. A pair of red and silver Kastle's—all mine. That ski park became my escape during the long, snowy Minnesota winters. I hadn't thought our neighborhood could achieve further greatness until Mount Villa came along. I'd trudge down Shryer in my boots, skis resting on my shoulder, then onto Dale Street, and after a quick right I was there. A lift ticket was a buck or less and my babysitting money more than covered it. The countless hours I spent skiing kept me out of trouble, at least during the winter months.

Life was good. I briefly experimented with the "bad crowd" in seventh grade, but in those days, "bad" hardly meant the same thing that it does today. We once discovered a stripped down mannequin in one of the dressing rooms in a Dayton's department store and yanked off its arms, concealing them in the sleeves of our jackets as we walked out of the store. My favorite was the right arm with its thumb and forefinger pointed like a gun. We stashed the arms in our school lockers and pulled them out between classes, shoving them up our long sleeved shirts and using them to point at random kids in the hallways. It was hysterical. Then during class I'd "raise my arm" and "point" at the blackboard. My teachers' exasperated expressions seemed to say, "why did I ever think teaching junior high kids was a good idea?" It wasn't until we later discovered that mannequins were expensive for retailers to buy and replace and that our theft might constitute a felony that some measure of guilt and fear set in.

I ultimately decided that type of delinquent behavior wasn't worth risking my long-term plans, so I started spending more time with my friends from the neighborhood and meeting new people. We were all typical suburban kids from working and middle class families during those wonderfully frightening years of experimentation and intense socialization. My friends were everything to me. Some my parents approved of, others not so much. But I liked to mix it up, so I knew which I could bring around and which had to remain "friends from school," assuring they'd most likely never meet my parents.

In April of 1972, my mom and dad celebrated their 25th wedding anniversary. At that point they were enjoying their five grandchildren. I remember Grandma Evelyn with her camera trying to capture a good picture of my nieces and nephews all together. She had me play the role of "herder," since I'd earned my herding credentials with Lisa and Eric. My father was still working in spite of his poor health.

We owned a small plot of land on Borden Lake in Garrison, Minnesota. We couldn't afford a cabin, but there was an outhouse, and we'd park our camper up there when we stayed. My parents talked a lot about what they were going to do with that property "someday." Funny how some dreams are never realized because the unexpected often thwarts our most hopeful of plans. That random turn of events came in the late summer of 1972, though it didn't seem that arbitrary to me. My grandmother Evelyn had predicted it would happen—it had just been a matter of time. By then, she'd so thoroughly reconstructed and catalogued my mother's family history she likely could have diagnosed her as well as any doctor. The only thing she didn't have was a name.

We were up at Borden Lake. A typical stifling summer weekend. Mom was involved in her usual routines, which looked like a bunch of tedious work to me: cooking breakfast, lunch, or dinner on the propane stove, hanging wet beach towels on the clothesline, helping my dad clean sunfish. I was expected to keep Lisa and Eric entertained, but occasionally I'd sneak into the small fishing boat and row out to the middle of the lake by myself—sometimes with a book, but usually just to be alone. I'd barely tied off the boat after one of those excursions when I discovered my parents rushing to pack up the car. I wasn't sure what was going on; it wasn't even Sunday yet. All I knew was that we had to leave right away. There was something wrong with Mom. She was bleeding and needed to see a doctor right away.

My mind raced back to the conversation I'd had with Grandma Evelyn a few years earlier. My mom's surgery had been in 1957; was this something related to that? I'd just assumed she'd been taking care of her health. But that hadn't been the case. For those fifteen or so years, she'd again avoided seeing any doctors other than for her pregnancies. The reason, according to my older sisters, was that she'd gained weight and didn't want to be called out by her doctors.

Suddenly, I felt very guilty. Guilty that I'd loved the fact that if I ever got lost in a store, I could quickly run down the aisles and spot my mom because she was heavy. Guilty that, knowing how cruel kids could be in the 4th grade, I grabbed a tray of homemade cupcakes—lovingly decorated with vanilla frosting and little rosebuds—from her in the hallway at Lexington Elementary the day of my class birthday celebration.

I told her, "Thanks," then shut my classroom door in her face so my classmates wouldn't see her. I couldn't handle the jokes and snide comments from my ten-year-old peers. The guilt crushed me. And now we were throwing the cooler and our soaked swimsuits into the station wagon as quickly as possible so we could rush her back to the Twin Cities; all because she'd gone into the outhouse and come out with a shocked look on her increasingly pale face.

Once home, the situation worsened. My mom was told she had advanced colon cancer and again needed immediate surgery, but this time she'd most likely end up with a total colectomy and colostomy bag. That was the *good* prognosis. Her surgeon, Dr. Schultz, was a handsome, Northwestern University-educated colorectal surgeon who had a direct, no-nonsense style we needed. I liked him the moment I met him. If I had to describe Dr. Schultz, I'd call him "swashbuckling" but with a surgeon's scalpel instead of a sword. His biggest concern at that time was that the cancer might have spread to my mom's liver.

I was approaching the start of eighth grade, and with my mom's health crisis, it looked like my extracurricular activities would be sharply curtailed. My brother Walt was on the high school football team but wasn't very committed given what was going on. He even blew off a game and hitchhiked several miles before being picked up by a family friend who took him to Midway Hospital where the surgery would take place.

My dad tried to assume both roles while Mom was in the hospital and later recovering from surgery, but he soon realized he needed my sister Marcie to help out. She was at the University of Minnesota studying business—a young woman declaring a business major was blasphemy in those days—and working at a furniture store trying to pay her way through college. She received no financial help from my parents despite living away from home at only twenty years old. Now she got to add "surrogate mother" to her routine. I remember coming home from school and Marcie would be there making dinner for us. It was almost always ham and corn, corn and ham— you'd think she could change the dinner options every now and then. Maybe a TV dinner or chicken pot pie like when I was a little kid, but no. We were a family adrift.

Not only was Marcie going to college, working part time, and taking care of us, she also took care of my mom when she returned home after the removal of her colon and a hysterectomy. Figuring the worst was over since Mom had survived the surgery and was back home, I tried to sneak out of the house one night in order to avoid kitchen duty. Just before I reached the door, Marcie shouted for me to come to my mom and dad's bedroom. *Too late*, I muttered under my breath, knowing I'd be in for the evening. I walked slowly, taking small, measured steps. Pleasant memories of my parents' bedroom flashed through my mind: rummaging through my mom's costume jewelry and trying on gleaming necklaces and bracelets in front of the antique mirror above her dresser; rifling through her dresser drawers looking for white gloves that would complement my Easter dress; playing dress-up in Mom's high heels while dabbing her perfume behind my ears. It was an inviting room to me as a child, but as I walked toward that bedroom I was terrified.

I stood in the doorway, not wanting to enter, not wanting to come too close. My mom lay in bed on her back, her stomach and post-surgical wound fully exposed. She kept her arm draped over her eyes as if she didn't want to see what was going on around her, or perhaps the look on my face. Marcie sat beside my mom and cleaned the area around her open wound with something that looked eerily like a turkey baster. I thought I might be sick.

Marcie looked up at me and said, "I might not always be able to come home to help with Mom's care, Laura, so I may need you to step in once in a while." She then showed me how to clean the stoma on her abdomen and asked if I had any questions. I lied and told her "no," anxious for it to be over. I felt my cheeks cool as the blood drained from them, and struggled to keep my face expressionless.

As might have been the thought of many thirteen-year-olds in similar circumstances, my only thought was, *How the hell am I going to hang out with my friends and ski at Villa if I have to be responsible for this?* It was as if that strong and thoughtful girl they'd known from a few years earlier had been replaced by a taller, more foul-mouthed, and self-centered whiny brat. *Oh God, this is too much for me*, I thought. *What about Walt? Can't he handle a turkey baster? Why can't he be the backup?* In my selfishness, I failed to consider that in my mother's state of dress and with her wound exposed, she would, of course, have preferred a female to take care of her. I wanted to tear my hair out and never thought about what might happen if my mother's cancer had metastasized to her lymph nodes or liver—we were still waiting for those tests to come back.

I stayed silent as I watched Marcie gently attach a new ostomy bag. I could never lash out and say what I was thinking—that would be too hurtful. I started to feel guilty, which took my mind off the bile pooling in my throat. Good thing our bathroom sink was just a few feet to the left to deposit the contents of my ham and corn dinner. But as bad as all of that was, it was about to get much worse.

Dr. Schultz encouraged my father to have all of the kids "checked out" as soon as possible. There was a strong likelihood that the problem my mother had could have been passed on to her kids. Without fanfare, we were systematically set up with Dr. Schultz for examinations of the lower part of our colon. Lisa and Eric were too young, but all the rest of us from Debbie on down to me wound up in his office for proctology exams or "proctos." I remember having to prep for my exam. Not exactly a normal thing for an eighth grader, but anything that got me out of algebra was okay with me. Better to prep for a colon exam than an algebra exam, even if it meant spending time in the bathroom fumbling with an enema bag.

Walt and I went to see Dr. Schultz together at his office in St. Paul. I don't remember who drove us to the appointment. I *do* remember that Walt went first. He didn't look happy when I passed him on my way into the office. He mouthed the words, "Just you wait," as I went. I suppose I should have been terrified, but I was pretty clueless about the procedure I was about to undergo. I didn't panic until I saw the scope—a long rigid tube—and immediately thought maybe algebra wasn't so bad after all.

Then Walt and I got "the news." I was clean, he wasn't. That's the terminology we used—your colon was either "clean" and therefore completely void of polyps, or not. And if it wasn't, there could be hundreds of them. Walt had multiple polyps growing inside of his colon, which were "markers" for what Dr. Schultz called a multiple polyposis syndrome. So did Debbie,

Karen, and Butch. Marcie was clean. We'd have to wait until
Lisa and Eric were older to learn which category they'd fall
into—they'd have to be at least twelve or thirteen before any
examinations could take place.

Back at the house, Walt had more on his mind than I did;
after all, I got the "you're good for now" clean colon bill of
health. He, along with Debbie, Karen, and Butch—all three
parents of young children—would almost certainly be facing
some kind of surgery. My mom was still waiting to hear if the
cancer had spread to other organs in her body. Dad broke down
to Marcie and admitted he was worried about paying the
inevitable medical bills. Even with the generous insurance plan
provided by the Bricklayer's Union there would likely be
uncovered expenses. I'm sure she listened but doubt she would
have been much help; she had her own finances to worry about.
And me? My instinct was to learn as much about this syndrome
as I could in the hopes of preventing my own future polyp
invasion.

Dr. Schultz was a busy surgeon but he always made time to
talk with us about the polyposis syndrome. I can remember
him encouraging me to "fire away" with my questions and
thinking, *Maybe if I don't ask them, it will all just go away.*
What we were told then was that our family had a disorder
called familial adenomatous polyposis (FAP). There were other
names for this condition: adenomatous familial polyposis,
adenomatous familial polyposis syndrome, and familial
multiple polyposis syndrome. We just referred to it as "the
curse" or our "pesky colons."

Dr. Schultz told us that the colon polyps typically start
showing up in an affected person in their teens and twenties.
There was no medical test to determine which kids might have

the polyposis syndrome, so diagnosis came only through a review of our family history and the dreaded, yet necessary, colonoscopies.

If the doctor found any suspicious polyps during the exam, they were removed immediately. Otherwise, the potential for them to become cancerous was significant. Without proper treatment (surgery and surveillance), virtually all people diagnosed with FAP develop colon cancer by their early forties. Dr. Schultz made it very clear to all of us how important keeping up with our appointments was to our ongoing care plan.

The four kids found to have the polyps in 1972 (Debbie, age twenty-four, Karen, age twenty-three, Butch, age twenty-two, and Walt, age sixteen) were advised to have bowel resections, also known as subtotal colectomies, to remove all but eighteen inches of their colons as soon as possible. That remaining eighteen inches would need to be checked every year, and if any concerning polyps were present, Dr. Schultz would burn or "snip" them and send them to a pathology lab for biopsies.

Eventually, we accepted this new reality and even had fun with it once in a while. My older sisters would sometimes put temporary tattoos on their backsides that read, "slippery when wet" and "do not enter" prior to their proctology exams. We never underestimated the stress-reducing power of juvenile humor. We also became adept at performing the required enemas and surviving the pre-exam diet of clear liquid and gelatin. We often joked about hating gelatin and made sure it never made it to the post-1972 Thanksgiving dinner table or family celebrations during the summers that followed. It became known as the "no Jell-O rule."

I didn't talk much about the syndrome outside of the family. I might have mentioned to a few of my closest friends that "there was something health-related we needed to deal with." They didn't ask many questions but knew my mother had a "bag" and that we had to have our colons examined more frequently than "normal" people. The prep and the actual procedure were hardly experiences that my friends could identify with, so I stayed pretty silent on the topic.

Baker-Miller-Christensen Polyposis of the Colon

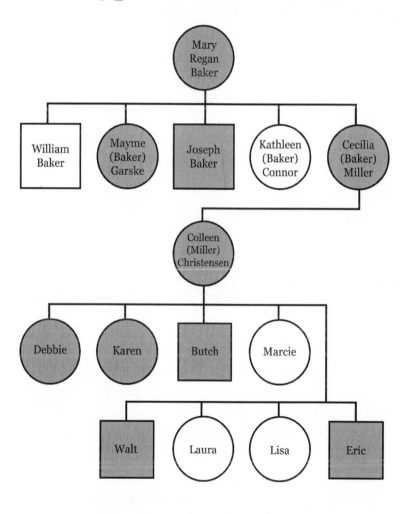

CHAPTER 6: FIND THE FAMILIES (1924-1970)

As early as the end of the nineteenth century, researchers had reported gastrointestinal syndromes that appeared to run in families. It's doubtful that any of these findings would have made their way into a public library in the late '40s and early '50s when my grandmother Evelyn was researching "summer's complaint," but she remained relentless in her pursuit of answers.

It's possible that my grandmother may have read about Dr. Cuthbert Dukes, an English physician, pathologist, and author affiliated with St. Mark's Hospital in London. He'd observed patients with a family history of colorectal cancer who presented with multiple adenomas of the colon likely to undergo malignant change. He named the disorder "polyposis." In 1924, after discovering a mutual interest in these families, Dukes and renowned surgeon J.P. Lockhart-Mummery established the first Polyposis Registry at St. Mark's Hospital.

Not only was Dr. Dukes a pioneer in the field of familial polyposis, his work stressed the importance of the family pedigree. He once stated that pedigrees in polyposis-prone families are like "photographs," which "record the state of affairs at a given point of time."

Decades later, in 1958, Dukes would publish his seminal report, "Cancer Control in Familial Polyposis of the Colon." At a presentation of his work at the Mayo Clinic in Rochester, Minnesota in October of 1958, he stated, "I have purposely entitled this paper, 'Cancer Control in Familial Polyposis of the Colon' because I shall confine myself almost exclusively to questions concerned with the prevention and early treatment of cancer in polyposis families. It would be difficult to find a more promising field for the exercise of cancer control than a polyposis family, because both diagnosis and treatment are possible in the precancerous stage and because the results of surgical treatment are excellent." Dukes believed that if a patient remained asymptomatic until the age of forty, it was very unlikely that they would develop polyps later.

At that time, genetics as a field of study was still in its infancy, and it would be decades more before it was well enough understood to make the critical connections necessary to diagnose our family and others with similar inherited disorders. Nonetheless, Dr. Dukes made the connection between his own research and the growing field of genetics, and penned this poetic vision of a future in which gene therapy for polyposis might be possible:

You are old, Father William, the young surgeon said,
And your colon from polyps is free.
Yet most of your siblings are known to be dead—
A really *bad* family tree.
In my youth, Father William replied with a grin,
I was told that a gene had mutated,

That all who carried this dominant gene
To polyps and cancer were *fated.*
I sought for advice from a surgical friend,
Who sighed and said—Without doubt
Your only escape from an untimely end
Is to have your intestine right *out.*
It seemed rather bad luck—I was then but nineteen—
So I went and consulted a quack,
Who took a firm grip on my dominant gene
And promptly *mutated it back.*
This, said the surgeon, is something quite new
And before we ascribe any merit
We must see if the claims of this fellow are true,
And observe what your *children* inherit!

Though unlikely, Evelyn may also have stumbled upon the British scientific weekly journal *Nature*, published on April 25, 1953 and read a one-page paper describing the findings of James Watson and Francis Crick entitled "A Structure for Deoxyribose Nucleic Acid." And even if she had, she may not have understood the significance of their discovery of the double helix—the twisted-ladder structure of deoxyribonucleic acid (DNA), which was a milestone in genetic science. Even after the discovery of the double helix, very little was known about the hereditary factors that contribute to human disease when my mother underwent her first subtotal colectomy in 1957.

As Eldon J. Gardner, an early researcher of cancer "clusters" in Utah families, expressed in his "Genetics of Cancer and Other Abnormal Growths" presentation as part of the Utah State University Faculty Honor Lectures series in the 1950s:

"The cancer problem will eventually be solved by the application of the scientific method. In fact, the solution may actually be very simple when the secret has been learned. Now it is extremely complex."

The complexity of the problem was vast, yet receiving funding for research was often difficult for those on the front lines working with families. Unfortunately, in the United States in the 1960s, the medical establishment wasn't always known to support the efforts of those early researchers studying inherited cancer syndromes.

As an Internal Medicine resident at the University of Nebraska College of Medicine in the 1960s, Dr. Henry T. Lynch met with many patients whose family members had been found to have the same or similar types of cancers that they themselves had been diagnosed with. Given his background in the burgeoning field of genetics, Dr. Lynch postulated that some of these cancers might have hereditary origins. This flew in the face of the long accepted belief in several American medical circles that cancer stemmed almost exclusively from environmental factors. Unrelenting, the idea that these cancers might be of hereditary origin became the main focus of Dr. Lynch's work in the 1960s and into the 1970s. His painstaking recordkeeping and meticulous compilations of family medical histories led him to identify a number of cancer syndromes and their patterns of inheritance through generations of extended Midwestern families.

In 1970—two years before my mother's cancer diagnosis would send six of her children to have their colons examined—Dr. Lynch applied for a National Institute of Health grant to study the phenomena in more depth. In his grant proposal, he presented the case of a family in which numerous members presented with colon cancer, though without the multiple polyps that had been identified as markers in FAP. He clearly showed that given the prevalence of colon cancer in the general population, there must have been some other factors at work to account for the increased pervasiveness within this singular family unit. Nevertheless, the committee reviewing his proposal did not agree and resoundingly rejected the notion that the cancers diagnosed in the families he'd been working with could solely be due to inherited factors. Some suggested that this unmitigated dismissal was rooted in a fear within the medical community that acknowledging cancer could have a genetic component would cause a panic.

Resolute in his convictions, Dr. Lynch continued to apply for many other grants and was, more often than not, rejected. Nevertheless, he continued his research on minimal funding and worked with these families and their primary doctors, convinced that he would one day be able to prove his hypothesis. Whether inherited cancer syndromes were considered too rare to justify funding, or because of concerns about how people might react to learning they carried a genetic mutation, generations of "cancer families" around the globe, including my own, continued to wait for answers.

CHAPTER 7: SAN FRANCISCO

1972 was a difficult year for our family, but it wasn't without things to be grateful for. My mom's cancer hadn't metastasized to her liver or lymph nodes or anywhere else as far as her test results showed. She and my siblings recovered from their surgeries; Walt went back to playing football for his high school team, and the others went back to living their lives and raising their young families.

In the spring of 1973, my mom suggested we drive out to the West coast for a summer vacation. Dad was always up for a road trip as long as he was behind the wheel, but the excursion she was thinking of included a stop to see her biological father in San Francisco.

So, while hanging around the Wilsons' front stoop after an afternoon of swimming, I mentioned to Kim and Linda that I'd be leaving town for a few weeks at the end of the month on a vacation with my family. I'd had my braces tightened that morning, and my teeth still hurt so San Francisco came out "Sanfisco." I wasn't thrilled with the idea of living out of a motor home for two weeks; it may as well have been a forced abduction, minus the handcuffs and duct tape.

I visualized myself behind the wheel of a Winnebago driving a stretch of open road in Arizona and mused, "It'd be cool if my dad lets me drive for a while. My mom drove tractors up on her family's farm when she was fourteen. Same thing."

The leg of the trip that worried me most was the stop to visit my grandfather Reggie and his wife, Olive, in California. I barely knew the man, but based upon a jumble of meager childhood memories, I'd never warmed up to either of them.

Perhaps my mom's cancer surgery the previous year had sparked some sort of longing in her to physically reconnect with her biological father again. Other than a few minutes of black and white footage in our family movies, Reggie and Olive didn't show up much, and when they did they always seemed to be waving goodbye. They never stayed with anyone—they were "hotel people." They may have stopped by our house once or twice when I was little, but that would have been it. While I could point him out in pictures, in an in-the-flesh line up, I might not even recognize my grandfather.

When my dad pulled the motor home into our driveway, I practically tore a hole in the screen door to be the first to check out my soon-to-be temporary living quarters. It had a green stripe with a big "W" on the side and was around twenty feet long. There was space with a mattress and a window that hung over the cab that I immediately claimed for the duration of the trip. There was a stove, a sink and refrigerator, and a table and benches that could be converted to a sleeping space. Best of all, there was a real bathroom in the back. Compared to camping in tents and the pop-up camper we pulled behind our station wagon on our last summer road trip, this was the lap of luxury.

I ran back into the house, found a piece of paper, a pen, and some scotch tape. I drew up a two-week calendar that included every day we'd be on the road, went back into the motor home, and climbed into space above the cab. I taped my crude calendar on the wall in anticipation of crossing off every day as we worked our way to California and back.

Once down on the floor of the camper, I opened the glove box and found what I was hoping to find—a fold out map of the US which included all the states and the major freeways and highways. I would need that to follow our trip from my space above the cab. I tucked it under my shirt and went back to the house to start packing.

On the road, Lisa and I jostled for position in our new digs. I'd agreed to share the upper space with her as long as she wasn't annoying. I alone would decide what constituted annoying. Over the intervening years, Lisa and I had developed our own special sibling rivalry—one that I thought might someday push our mom over the edge. Lisa was afraid of the dark and wanted the door to our shared bedroom open to let light in from the hall. I, on the other hand, demanded complete darkness and exacerbated her fears by telling her there were voices coming from the closet. Night after night, my mom had to deal with the inevitable drama. Lisa took her revenge by spying on my friends and me, which drove me equally crazy.

As I kicked my sneakers off and climbed up next to her, I couldn't help but grin at a humorous memory. One Christmas when we were kids—and utilizing my burgeoning detective skills—I discovered that the brown, plainly-wrapped package stashed in my parent's bedroom closet was a doll Lisa had asked Santa to bring her. I matched the series of numbers on the outside of the rectangular-shaped package to the item number in the Sears Roebuck Christmas catalog. I'd already figured out that Santa and the Easter Bunny didn't exist, but at four-and-a-half years old, Lisa still didn't have a clue. Imagine her horror as I took her by the hand and revealed what I'd found. Not only had I guiltlessly spoiled her Christmas surprise, she too then knew that Santa wasn't real.

I had packed a huge stack of magazines—Tiger Beat, Glamour, and Mademoiselle. I figured Lisa, at twelve, could handle the latter two, and she'd like the posters of teen heartthrobs in Tiger Beat that she could tear out and tape to her bedroom wall upon our return. I, on the other hand, was looking forward to the "summer makeover" articles and makeup and exercise tips in the fashion magazines. After all, I'd soon be returning to Parkview for my final year of junior high with a mouthful of metal, so I needed to pay attention to things like making sure I wore the right eye shadow—brown, I learned, would make my blue eyes "pop" as I strutted down the halls. With my older sisters all out of the house, those magazines were my only hope of avoiding a dreaded fashion faux pas and worse, potential social irrelevance.

We were taking a never-been-traveled southwestern route through Missouri, down into Oklahoma on I40, and across the Texas panhandle. From there we'd drive into New Mexico and then Arizona where we planned to stop for a few days at Grand Canyon National Park. I was particularly excited about that leg of the trip. Up until that point, I'd only seen pictures in National Geographic magazines; the majestic photographs imprinted on my brain for years. It was everything I'd hoped it would be. Stopping at a popular lookout at the south rim, the pink and blue hues of the canyon became layers of vibrant purple and red. The sheer size and splendor of this natural treasure made me gasp. It was magnificent. I imagined I felt a bit like Neil Armstrong had a few years earlier when he first stepped out of Apollo 11 onto the moon. My dad, his own curiosity piqued, bought me a book about the national park written by a notable historian. It made for absorbing reading in my space above the cab as our road trip continued.

Seven hours and nearly 500 miles after we pulled out of our Arizona campsite and over 2,000 miles from home, we arrived in Anaheim, California. I'd begged my parents to stay at least one or two nights in a hotel so we could have access to a swimming pool. Disneyland was also on the docket. The hotel wasn't much, but it was next door to an all-you-can-eat buffet-style Chinese restaurant, which was a bonus. It was cooler than normal (62 degrees in the afternoon sun), but that didn't stop us from jumping into the pool.

People walked past asking, "Are you kids crazy? Aren't you freezing?"

We'd reply, "Nope, we're from Minnesota." Then they'd smile and nod their heads, understanding completely.

My dad filmed us with his Super 8 while we splashed and waved. He also caught me at the deep end of the pool treading water while waiting for Eric to come down the slide. I was supposed to catch him. For some reason I was momentarily distracted, and Eric splashed down without me. I quickly swam over and grabbed him to help him keep his head above water. Lisa was laughing. I was laughing. Eric wasn't laughing. I won his trust again the next day at Disneyland by accompanying him and Lisa on the little kid rides. In the pictures my parents took of us that day, I'm not smiling. Maybe it was the embarrassment of my new braces, or it could have been the fact they were taking pictures of me on lame rides. Or maybe I was just too old for Bear Country, the Tiki Room, and "It's a Small World."

The drive from Los Angeles to San Francisco was uneventful except for a brief stop off the 101 to visit a town called Solvang. Solvang was a town of Danish immigrants and everyone we met was a Petersen or an Olsen, a Christensen or an Andersen. Some variation of "-sen." My dad enjoyed a Danish pastry, which he declared "as authentic as the ones his mother brought home from the local Scandinavian bakery." I smiled at my dad, picking up on the obvious jab at my Grandma Evelyn's lack of baking talent. That small town was so different from the bustle of southern California, and I felt very comfortable there in that tiny slice of "Denmark." Back on the road and heading north, we managed to find Reggie and Olive's place without any problems. We parked the camper in the driveway of their home, which was not too far from Fishermen's Wharf and the Pacific Ocean—the two "must-do's" on my list.

We left our things in the camper and walked up the concrete steps toward the front door. My grandfather must have seen us from the big picture window as we pulled into the driveway—he opened the door before my mom reached for the doorbell. My first thought was that he looked much older than I was expecting. It was as if we were meeting for the first time. He was in his late 60s according to my mom, but looked as if he was well into his 70s. His hug felt obligatory and stilted. This was no joyous, tearful reunion. Olive was wearing a dress and had loads of jewelry hanging from her neck and wrists—gaudy stuff that nonetheless looked like the real thing—extravagances my mother would never have been able to afford. She still wore the same cat-eye style glasses I remembered from the old black and white photos, and smelled of Tabu (*the forbidden fragrance*) and cigarette smoke.

I knew we were only going to be visiting for a few days, but even that suddenly seemed interminable. The house was perfectly clean—no dust anywhere, nothing out of place. Even the mirror above the wet bar in the dining room was spotless. The house positively screamed "no kids." I noticed a book of matches with my grandfather's picture on the front. *Figures*, I thought to myself. Working my way down the hallway, I spotted a room that looked to be a den with a color television on. I motioned for Lisa and Eric to follow me and heard Olive say something like, "I bet you kids are hungry. Let me see what I can find."

"Sure," I said under my breath, "like the kitchen?" She didn't hear me, but Eric and Lisa burst out laughing.

I was playing with the dials on the TV when I heard raised voices coming from the other room. My mom and Reggie were in the midst of a heated disagreement. I gave Lisa and Eric the "shush" signal, but before I could eavesdrop, Olive appeared in the doorway.

"Chop chop," she said, clapping her hands together. "Here's some money for you to go to McDonald's for lunch. There's one not too far from here. Laura, you're in charge." She pressed a dollar bill and some change into my outstretched right hand.

A buck seventy-five? Are you kidding me? I thought. *I bet Lisa has more money in her plastic Minnie Mouse wallet. Have you even been to a McDonald's?* I closed my fist around the cash and marched into the living room. Fortunately, on our way out, my dad slipped me a five-dollar bill. He must have seen the look of frustration on my face.

I left the house with Lisa and Eric to find the McDonald's. I was smart enough to jot down Reggie and Olive's address in case we got lost. We had no map, no idea where to go, and were in a big city far from home. And hungry.

Great goddamn start to San Fran, I grumbled to myself.

We must have looked ridiculous wandering around the neighborhood asking people if they could point us to the McDonald's. We walked for over an hour.

"This is a bunch of shit!" I exclaimed and gave Eric a don't-tell-mom-and-dad-I-swore-in-front-of-you look. I still owed him one after failing to catch him in the pool, so I figured the odds of him tattling on me were no better than fifty-fifty.

Eventually, we did find the McDonald's; we all had shakes with our food and then managed to find our way back to Reggie and Olive's antiseptic home just in time to interrupt cocktail hour. A bottle of gin and another of tonic water was on the console. My parents sat shoulder to shoulder on the couch paging through a photo album while my mom reminisced about her summers in Devils Lake. Everyone was all smiles and laughter, the argument from earlier apparently forgotten.

We all managed to remain on our best behavior for Reggie and Olive until we left San Francisco. There were no tears shed when we departed, just as there had been none when we arrived. I would miss that fantastic city and the house with its big picture window—my grandfather and his bossy wife not so much. I intuitively understood that the visit was something that my mom needed. I hoped she found what she'd been looking for. All I found was the realization that I was outgrowing road trips with my family—and that damned McDonald's.

CHAPTER 8: WORKING THE PLAN

I started high school in the fall of 1974, a little over a year after our San Francisco adventure. The worst part was leaving those friends that would be attending the rival high school in our city, Frank B. Kellogg. Parkview was split—half the kids moved on to Alexander Ramsey High School and the other half were sent to Kellogg. It was a teenage travesty. Worse, the geographic dividing line that determined which students went to which high school was Dale Street—literally at the end of the road I lived on. My boyfriend at the time, along with many of my friends from Parkview, went to Kellogg. I wound up at Ramsey. I think I suffered from borderline clinical depression in tenth grade over this random existential catastrophe that had split up my peer group. Eventually, I passed my driver's test, and my dad bought me an old but dependable '65 Oldsmobile that shuttled me, Linda, Kim, and Toree to school, Burger Chef for lunch, and Kellogg whenever we had sixth-hour study hall.

While at Ramsey, I played the part of the good student and obedient teenager well, just as I had done in grade school and junior high. I joined the yearbook staff and took advantage of the ski club with my fellow Mount Villa conquerors, Patti and Joann. More critically, I maintained a solid GPA so my parents left me alone. But I also had a fake ID that I used to sneak into the local bars where the college kids hung out. Had they found out, my parents would never have believed it, and as long as I didn't come home smelling like cigarettes or liquor in the middle of the night and kept my grades up, I could talk my way out of pretty much any transgression.

In 1975, my father had to retire on total disability. For years, he'd needed a cane and had difficulty standing from a seated position. During that time, I often accompanied him to the store to catch the change that would inevitably slip through his gnarled, arthritic fingers. That proud man hated the fact that he was dependent on others for the simple activities of daily living. He never said so out loud, but I knew.

We now qualified for reduced-cost lunch tickets at Ramsey, which was also embarrassing for my father. He was extremely upset when I told him there was a separate line for the "discounted lunch ticket kids." Lisa was the only one who had to stand in that line, because I either didn't eat, drove to a local place to grab lunch, or left school early in the afternoon to go to my job. It bothered my dad so much that I offered to stand in the "poor kids" line for Lisa and give her the months' worth of lunch tickets to save her from the embarrassment. I didn't care how it looked. In fact, I would have stood in line for any of those kids if asked. But the question remained—what kind of idiot thought it was a good idea to separate kids out by income in front of their peers? I was lucky in that my group of high school friends came from diverse economic backgrounds and family situations. I never felt poor, but I did shoulder much of the same financial insecurity that plagued my parents. Those health problems we didn't always see coming could clean out a savings account in a heartbeat.

I remember a fight my parents had one night not long before I graduated from high school. They really never fought much, so this one surprised me. My father was furious that my mom had taken $428 out of a savings account my Auntie Del had set up to help pay for my college. I'd known that account had been drained for years. I assumed my mom needed the money to pay medical bills, which is what she was trying to explain to my dad. He wasn't having any of it. It was hard enough for him knowing he wouldn't be able to help me with college, but finding out that what little we did have was gone, made it that much worse. Their arguing escalated until finally I couldn't take it anymore. I'd been fortunate to find a job with the State Job Service Office that allowed me to work full time over summer breaks and part time during the school year, and had put away nearly every paycheck for college. I stormed into the living room and told them to knock it off because I'd already saved enough to cover tuition and books. I said I didn't want to hear any more about the missing money. They fell silent and looked at me with a mixture of surprise and relief. And they never brought it up again.

When high school was finally over, I granted my mom's wish and wore a dress to graduation. *Who'd see it under my gown anyway?* I thought. Over time, that little first-grader who'd adored the checkered dress with the embroidered leaves on its white collar had turned into a tomboy. My mom would say my fashion sense devolved into hippie-meets-militaristic— leather fringed vests and green army fatigues.

In the fall I was off to the University of Minnesota. I shared a first-floor apartment with two much older roommates who often provided big sister-like advice about my late-night study habits and strange diet. I survived on gallons of coffee, condensed soup, and dehydrated mashed potatoes. My faithful Oldsmobile stayed with my parents—insurance would have been an impossible expense—so I rode my bike or took the bus to campus. I was suddenly and completely financially independent from my parents, and though money was a constant consideration, it was a liberating and exhilarating experience. My success (or failure) was all on me. It felt fantastic, even when I occasionally stumbled along the path of my plan. But there was also considerable pressure to succeed— both of my own making and from my parents. They wanted more for me academically than they'd been able to achieve, and they pushed me as hard as I pushed myself.

My first two years in a college setting were unremarkable. I did well in the classes I liked (English composition, humanities, history) and not so well in those I was required to take as part of my "generals" (astronomy, geology). I lucked out in that I was in one of the last graduating classes at the U that could substitute a philosophy class for my math credit requirement. Once I hit my major (Communications), my classes became more interesting, and my focus on the future sharpened.

I was also fortunate to find an on-campus job with the Virology Lab in Jackson Hall. The money was better than any off-campus job I could find, and it paid my rent and grocery bill so I didn't have to dip into my savings. Plus, I worked side by side with some brilliant women who were medical lab techs; even the lab manager was a woman who'd worked as a nurse for many years. My job was clerical, but I understood their roles in identifying viruses found in cultures and determining through blood serology whether or not someone had a certain level of immunity to things like the measles and chicken pox. I thought their jobs were very interesting—mine not so much. I was tasked with running a metal basket around the U's hospital and various clinics picking up specimens, which might be anything from urine to chunks of tissue. I'd bring them back to the lab and log them into the appropriate "database," which at that time was nothing more than a three-ring binder. At first, handling the specimens made me queasy, but over time I pushed through it and started asking my lab co-workers questions. What is Cytomegalovirus? Are viruses capable of causing the development of human cancers? What happens if you are infected with Epstein Barr virus? Given my experience with a familial cancer syndrome, I had a million questions. My position at the lab allowed me access to people who might be able to help me understand the underlying science of our disease in a safe setting where there were no stupid questions. They tolerated me well.

Right around that same time, one of Karen's daughters was admitted to Methodist Hospital in Minneapolis for some kind of benign jaw tumor. It was bony, and she complained it hurt and woke her up at night as she moved her head around on her pillow. She was about ten years old at the time. I drove to Methodist to visit her. When I walked into her room I found her sitting up in bed combing the hair on a stuffed animal, while a cup of clear soup sat uneaten on a bedside tray. My sister Karen filled me in. The doctors weren't overly concerned, but they did want to find a way to reduce the tumor's size or remove it so she would be more comfortable. They thought she might have some kind of juvenile arthritis, which made sense to me since my dad suffered from severe rheumatoid arthritis for years. I thought maybe that disease could also run in families. After minor surgery and a short stay, she was sent home and fully recovered from the jaw issue, but strangely, she never complained about having arthritic joint pain the way my father did.

While at the University, I took a course called "Heredity and Human Society" as a junior to fulfill a science requirement. My real motivation for signing up for that class was that I didn't have to take a lab with it. Plus, a couple of guy friends from my junior high days were also taking the course. The three of us sat in the back row of the lecture hall and took notes for one another in case any of us missed class.

We had fun in that class, especially when the topic turned to what sexually transmitted diseases could do to human genitals. Those pictures up on the big screen in the lecture hall scared the hell out of us. The professor was a big, strong gentleman by the name of Val. He appeared to be part Native American, and his seductive baritone kept my rapt attention.

The "heredity" part of the class began with the usual Mendelian pea pod experiments I'd learned about in high school biology.

Gregor Mendel was an Australian monk widely considered to be the founder of the modern science of genetics. Mendel's pea plant experiments conducted between 1856 and 1863 established many of the basic rules of heredity, now referred to as the laws of Mendelian inheritance. He published his work in 1866, demonstrating the actions of invisible "factors"—now called genes—in providing predictability for the inheritance of certain physical traits.

When we moved away from plants and onto inherited diseases in humans, I began to pay closer attention. We learned that some human diseases are inherited in the same predictable pattern as in Mendel's experiments, because they also result from specific differences in single genes. Our cells use our genes as a blueprint to build and maintain our bodies, and just as is true with plants, we inherit one copy of each gene from our mother and one from our father. Having one bad or "mutated" copy of a gene could be catastrophic, or it could be inconsequential. It all depends on what the gene does (or does not) code for. As an example, if a person inherits a non-functional copy of a gene that would otherwise code for a piece of important cellular machinery—let's say to break down a toxin—the cell will just use the good copy to pick up the slack. Two bad copies, however, result in toxin buildup and manifests as illness. This scenario describes a form of "recessive genetic disorder," wherein disease occurs only in people who've inherited two bad copies of the gene, but a healthy person with one bad copy acts as a "silent carrier," allowing the disease—but not the gene—to skip generations.

Dominant genetic disorders, on the other hand, can be thought of as the result of a "troublemaker"—a gene with a blueprint for destruction. In this scenario, only one bad copy is needed to mess up part of the cellular machine, regardless of what the good copy is able to do. In this scenario, gene and disease are one and the same, and only offspring lucky enough to inherit two good copies are spared.

It dawned on me sitting there in class that that was exactly what had happened with my family. My mother had been an only child who carried a bad gene for a colon cancer pre-disposition syndrome, and she'd passed it on to at least four of her eight children. I closed my eyes and saw the squares and circles that were my sisters and brothers as I visualized our very own pedigree chart. When I opened my eyes to focus back on the screen in the lecture hall, Larry had written, "Are you OK?" on my notebook. I wasn't sure.

Does Mom know about any of this? I wondered. Later that day, just after dinner, I dropped the bombshell on her. I didn't do it to be cruel, but instead to point out something relevant I'd learned in class that day. I sat at the kitchen table with a cup of coffee in hand and blurted, "Mom, do you realize that you polluted the gene pool?" I explained that as an only child, she'd had the opportunity to prevent a mutated gene for a predisposition to colon cancer from ever being passed on. In having eight children, a condition that could have "ended," had instead been handed down to at least four of her kids and possibly her grandkids.

She didn't say much standing at the sink and was probably happy that I was paying attention in class. But I know my words hurt her. She didn't fight back. She didn't state the obvious: that if she'd decided not to have kids, I wouldn't be sitting there at that moment, a mouthy, smart-ass young woman accusing her of mucking up our hereditary line. *None of us* would be around. She also didn't point out that we'd all been born prior to the availability of birth control pills. She just listened to me spout off and continued to busy herself in the kitchen. Initially, it felt good to get that important information off my chest. But once I'd finished reciting all the facts and statistics that I'd learned from my Heredity and Human Society lecture that day, I didn't feel very good about it at all. What she didn't say in her silence was that at the time she was raising her young family and the field of medical genetics was evolving, there was no way she could have known.

During my spring quarter in 1980, I was in the Coffman Union student center at the University one night going over some homework assignments for a Theories of Interpersonal Communication class. I was looking for a distraction, so I bought a local newspaper and a coffee drink the University had recently introduced called a "cappuccino." I remember thinking, *This concoction has* definite *potential.* The paper contained the usual local "kitten stuck in a tree" news I used to vilify, but an article on the back page of the Metro section caught my eye. It was about how "freckles" found on the retina were an apparent marker for a syndrome that predisposed affected people to developing colon cancer called Familial Adenomatous Polyposis. Remarkably, as reported in the 1980 Journal of Ophthalmology, the same polyposis syndrome plaguing my family could also potentially be identified in a person via a simple eye exam, provided the optometrist or ophthalmologist knew what to look for.

I'd recently moved back home to save money, and, feeling empowered, I tossed the newspaper into the brown, faux suede book bag my mom had sewn for me, anxious to share it with my family. I already had plans to cut the article out and take it with me to my next eye appointment. It would be worth sharing, and might eventually prove to be just as effective and far less invasive than a colonoscopy.

Intrigued by this discovery, I made copies for each of my siblings in the student bookstore but not before stopping at the Virology Lab, excited to share the article with my co-workers. I had *a lot* of questions for them. Chief among them was whether or not I could skip future colonoscopies if I didn't have the freckling in my eyes. I was hopeful that this simple, non-invasive test might eliminate the need for those damn enema bags and proctoscopes.

PART TWO:

*Markers &
Moments*

CHAPTER 9: **WELCOME TO ADULTHOOD**

By the spring of 1982, my University of Minnesota days were behind me, and I entered the "early careerist" stage of life. The early to mid-'80s brought a lot of changes for my family and me. Despite a recession and a terrible job market for new college graduates, I was hired as an Employment Coordinator at the local office of Marsh and McLennan, Inc., a global property/casualty insurance brokerage firm. I remember the first time my dad came down to visit me at work. We were going to lunch together at the Foshay Tower. Our front desk receptionist walked him back to my office, and the look on his face said it all: *Cripes almighty, my daughter has her own private office.* He was so proud of me. For me, that office was the culmination of sticking to and accomplishing my plan. I'd managed to stay focused on school and finished what I'd set out to accomplish—to not have my script written for me as a teenager.

My parents had some incredible and unexpected good fortune around this time as well. In the eighties, a person could still buy stock in a small company without having to be "qualified." My dad took a little bit of money he'd saved (it helped that most of the kids had grown up and moved out by then) and bought stock in a medical device company called St. Jude after studying their annual reports and the other information available to a small investor. Over the course of a few years, he'd earned some sizable returns. Not that he was suddenly wealthy, but it was enough to buy new carpet for our living room (finally replacing the one we'd scorched with fiery marshmallows as kids) and new furniture. He and my mother and their friends from Faith Lutheran went on a cruise together—the first time my mom ever flew on an airplane. They were enjoying each other's company and that of their twelve grandchildren; I was so happy for them.

My dad's arthritis, however, was brutal and relentless. Despite knee replacements and experimentation with different medications to alleviate his joint pain, he still often required as many as eight anti-inflammatory painkillers a day to push through. His doctor would tell my mom, "I've never seen a guy in so much pain with such a positive attitude."

One evening I stopped by my parents' house to chat with my dad. He was considering flying to Mexico for an experimental shot that might help alleviate his pain, and I wasn't entirely comfortable with the idea. My ten-year-old niece sat on the front step wearing her team jersey with a softball in one hand and her glove on the other. She had a large bandage on her shin.

"Hey you," I said, nodding toward her leg. "Did you get smacked by a line drive?"

She gave me a wave and an engaging smile. "No, I had some stupid cyst removed."

"Was it bothering you?" I asked.

"Not really, but the doctor sliced it off anyway. I hope I don't have to slide into third tonight."

I tousled her hair. "Let me guess. You missed school today because of it, but you're still planning to play in the game tonight. You learn this kind of stuff from your Uncle Eric?"

She grinned sheepishly. "It's not that bad," she said.

My return home during my junior year of college to save money had allowed me to spend more time with my brother Eric during his high school years. We had some good talks—the type only an older sister can have with a teenage brother. He was a big help to my parents, especially my father, who needed a lot of help with the garden and other chores that needed to be taken care of around the house.

As we'd predicted, Eric was turning out to be an all-around great kid. He was a teenager, however, and wasn't immune to some of the typical predicaments teens fall into during their high school years. I remember coming home one night while my parents were out of town and, after seeing me pull into the driveway, Eric sheepishly opened the door and asked for my help "cleaning up after a party." I rescued him of course, but gave him a stern big sister mini-lecture as well. He'd already expressed a desire to become a police officer, and I explained that there were just some kinds of trouble he wouldn't want to have to disclose when applying for the law enforcement college program he hoped to attend. I think he appreciated my advice, and in turn didn't give me a hard time when I tossed his white football pants in the laundry with a load of jeans. There was a game that night, and it was too late to fix them, but he never said a word. It certainly wasn't hard for us to spot him on the field that night in those baby blue pants. And he played both offense and defense, so they saw a lot of playing time. What a trooper. And I'll never forget driving to Hurley, Wisconsin to go skiing at Indianhead Resort with Eric, Marcie, and her husband not long after Eric had turned eighteen. After a long day of wet and sloppy spring skiing we ended up at a local bar. As we hovered near the dance floor, Eric kindly whispered in my ear, "Could you please go stand somewhere else so I can pick up some girls to dance with?" Nothing like having your two big sisters looking over your shoulder to keep you out of the kind of trouble you're *trying* to get into.

I met Bill, the man who would become my husband, in early 1980, and he quickly became part of the family. Initially, I wasn't sure if Bill and I would even survive our first date. He took me to a nice restaurant with a Polynesian theme. We sat at a table for two in front of a tiny stage. During the live show I was pulled from the audience to go up and hula dance and be a good sport while playfully being made fun of. *Good thing I had a few of those fruity alcoholic drinks,* I thought, trying to hide my embarrassment. I must have taken it like a champ, because he asked me out again.

Eric cornered Bill to play catch the first time they met. After a few chucks of the baseball, Bill suggested football—his game. He'd been a wide receiver in high school and college. Like a couple of gladiators, they demonstrated their athletic prowess for one another, and Eric finally gave his blessing to his sister's new boyfriend by saying, "You've got a great arm."

Everyone liked Bill. He seemed "stable," they said. He had a good job, a reliable car, and had graduated from St. Thomas with a business degree. My mother, especially, took a shine to Bill and jumped at every opportunity to cook for him. Not only did he love her cooking, but his mother had died when he was only two years old so they were kindred spirits in that regard— motherless as young children. And they both loved animals.

My sisters, brothers, and I continued our colon exams as advised by Dr. Schultz. Marcie, Lisa, and I continued to present polyp-free, but Eric wasn't so fortunate. He joined the ranks of the siblings in the family who had the polyposis syndrome and required a subtotal colectomy as a young adult. Like the thoughtful young man he was, he scheduled his surgery so as not to interfere with his baseball team's busy summer schedule. He was their starting catcher and wanted to make sure he'd be able to complete the season. He asked me if he might end up with a colostomy bag like our mom. I tried to reassure him that the surgery should go well, but I was honest with him about the potential for colon cancer and the possibility of a future colostomy. But we all faced that risk, especially the siblings who knew they were most likely carriers of the familial polyposis syndrome. By then, Marcie had passed Dr. Schultz's milestone age of twenty-five with no polyps and I was nearly there, but that didn't mean we were in the clear—it just meant we could space our exams out over longer intervals.

There were advantages to all of us seeing the same colorectal surgeon. Not only was Dr. Schultz able to compare our exam results, he was also able to see how our personalities and attitudes helped us cope with a condition that we collectively needed to stay on top of. And he could leverage us against one another, encouraging a sibling-style peer pressure to make sure we didn't miss our appointments.

For those with the disorder, it was a bit like living with a ticking time bomb inside of them, with a timer no one could see.

The specter of living with a medical condition that could change course at any time didn't prevent me from wanting marriage and children, even though concerns remained about the polyposis syndrome. There was still no genetic test available at that time, so there was no way to be sure. Diagnosis relied almost exclusively on physical examination of the colon, and now the freckle on the retina tossed in as an additional marker. Bill knew about this when he asked me to marry him at Christmastime in 1983. It was a leap of faith for both of us.

In anticipation of our July wedding, my mother offered to sew my bridal gown. I was thrilled, because not only would I wear a dress sewn by my mother, it saved me the hassle and expense of trying to find one. I picked a dropped waist style with a somewhat plain skirt but with a heavily beaded bodice and long sleeves. When I told her I didn't mind if she glued the beads on the bodice of the dress, she nearly fainted. Only "cheap" wedding dresses had glued-on beads, according to my mom. And she was serious about this. She carried the bodice of my wedding dress, the beads, and a sewing needle and thread in a plastic bag everywhere she went for several months. While babysitting the grandkids, while waiting for my Dad at the doctor's office, even sitting in church. Any moment of downtime that presented an opportunity to sew on a few more beads, she went for it.

It was our kind of wedding. Short ceremony, a limited number of attendants, good food, and a rock band. With the help of family and friends, it all came together perfectly. Mom handled the dress, and Bill's stepmom took care of the flowers.

My friend Sarah picked out and performed the music. Despite the heat and humidity of a typical summer evening in Minnesota, the stars aligned on July 20, 1984, and we began our future together.

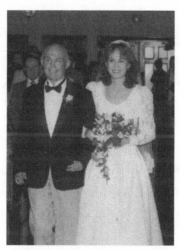

Dad walking me down the aisle

Upon returning from our honeymoon, I learned that my boss had turned in her resignation and Bob, our Head of Office, asked me to take on her role in an interim basis. I said yes, thrilled with the idea of becoming a Director and having responsibility for a budget and staff of my own. Around that same time, Bill had also been promoted to District Manager with American Express. We fell into an easy and comfortable work-life rhythm.

Summer turned to fall and fall to winter. My parents had booked a trip to Florida in early 1985 with their friends Rita and Fred; they returned in late February. Mom was glad to be back home because Dad had experienced some trouble while they were gone—he'd been complaining of shortness of breath while walking. It had become so concerning that the three of them had taken turns pushing him around Epcot in a wheelchair. Once home, he set up an appointment right away. Whatever his doctor's internist heard through the stethoscope must have been concerning, because he admitted my father to Midway hospital for "observation" that very day—a Wednesday or Thursday, I believe. Dad had a frequent visitor in my sister Lisa who lived with her husband, Mark, just a few blocks from the hospital. Lisa and Mark had gotten married the previous October, three months after Bill and I were married. I felt better knowing she was close by.

Then a once-in-a-decade blizzard hit. The snow started coming down hard on Friday, March 1, and by the weekend, travel was impossible. The Department of Transportation put out a bulletin—stay indoors and off the roads. My mom couldn't even back out of her driveway and wouldn't be able to for days. By Sunday, I convinced my sister-in-law to drive us to the hospital to see him, taking advantage of her four-wheel drive Subaru, the only weather-worthy car in the family that might be able to make the trip. I was worried because the doctors were supposed to see him and order tests the following day, but because of the storm, they were going to have to push those tests to Tuesday at the earliest.

When I arrived home, barely able to trudge up our driveway through the deep drifts of snow, I called my mother. "He doesn't seem himself," I told her. "He isn't watching TV or even reading the newspaper... He talked a lot about you and us kids." I didn't tell her that he glanced nervously at his heart monitor every few minutes. The whole day had so exhausted me I went to bed early. It was about 10:00 p.m., and I was staring up at the ceiling in the dark, thinking. Bill was lying next to me, but I wasn't sure if he was asleep. I looked down at the foot of our bed. There stood my father gazing down at me. He had a big smile across his face. His gnarled hands were gone, replaced by strong, healthy hands. He looked young again, like the man I'd once seen in the family movies—the handsome guy with the easy grin that my older brothers and sisters remembered as young children.

Terrified, I squeezed my eyes closed, opening them again only when I heard the sound of Lisa's frantic voice piped through our answering machine speakers. I felt the bed shift as Bill picked up the phone. I lay motionless on the bed and stared up at the ceiling, hoping it was all a bad dream, but the heat of the tears on my cheeks told me I was awake. I heard Bill speaking in hushed tones, but mostly he was quiet. Lisa was doing most of the talking. After a moment he set the phone down quietly and turned to me.

I already knew what he was going to say.

My father was gone.

CHAPTER 10: **SEEK AND YOU WILL FIND**

Some things just can't be explained. Or maybe they can be, but they don't make sense because you're too depressed to talk about it with anyone who can help you to understand. For instance, how does a fifty-five-year-old man with relatively few risk factors suddenly die in a hospital bed from a massive heart attack? Or, why was there a blizzard on the very weekend we all should have been at my dad's side? What about my father's apparition at the foot of my bed at the very moment he died?

We did learn that rheumatoid arthritis could eventually damage internal organs, and that the drugs my dad used to reduce the pain and inflammation are not good to be on long-term. But we were still in shock. My brother Eric was barely twenty-one years old—too young to lose a father. But one way or another, once the post-funeral luncheon dishes are cleared, people have to return to their routine. My family was no exception.

I threw myself into work that first week back, but wore sunglasses during the day because I didn't want anyone looking into my eyes. Eventually the shades went in one of my desk drawers, still in easy reach in case I was having a bad day. My boss and co-workers were great about giving me space and asking me how my family was doing.

I slogged my way through the spring and summer. By August, it was time for my annual performance review. This was more important than usual because we'd be talking about the possibility of my interim promotion becoming permanent and with it, the potential for an attractive salary increase.

Bob had a big corner office overlooking Nicollet Mall in downtown Minneapolis. A massive cherry wood desk and high-back leather chair that swiveled. Pictures of his family sat atop the matching cherry wood credenza. I felt small sitting in the chair across from him. The review went exceptionally well. He told me he was proud of the job I'd done and wanted me to stay in the position. I smiled and, of course, accepted. He'd recommended a nice pay increase for me, bringing me above the minimum range for my new management position.

When we were finished, we both signed the review. I stood and shook his hand. I told him how much I enjoyed working with him and thanked him for being so supportive. I was more than a little bit uncomfortable to drop the bomb on him.

I didn't have to wait long for his response. He rose from his chair and gave me a huge hug. As he pulled away, he said, "Congratulations, Laura. Being a parent is one of the greatest joys in my life, and you're going to make a great mother."

Alexander James was born in late February of 1986, the first grandchild born following my father's death, and almost to the day. He was two-and-a-half weeks past his due date. The "baby pool" at Marsh and McLennan had run out of gamblers. I remember teetering around in my heels fourteen days after he was due and hearing the exasperation in the voices of my mostly male co-workers, "You're still here? I lost twenty bucks on you!" My friend Mary, who worked in the property/casualty department, told me to ignore their ribbing, and said, "by the way, castor oil always worked for my mom." She'd come from a family of ten and that made her advice credible in my book.

I'd hoped the hospital Chaplain would stop by my room for a visit while I was there. Pastor Al was married to Kathy, another friend and colleague of mine at Marsh. I asked Kathy if he might be available to meet with me.

"Of course," she said, "I'll let him know you'd like a visit."

The day after Alex was born, Pastor Al—all lanky six feet three inches of him—peeked his head into my hospital room. "Hi Laura, Kathy mentioned you wanted to talk with me. Is now a good time?"

"Yes, please come in and grab a chair," I said. "I'm so happy you could stop by, I know you're a busy guy."

He pulled the only chair in the room next to my bed and leaned in. "How are you? Did everything go okay with you and your new son?"

"Oh, yes. Quite the adrenaline rush, this whole childbirth thing." Al was always easy to talk to.

As if he were reading my mind, he said, "This isn't about you or the baby, is it?"

I laughed. "No, not really. I just wanted to ask you a question or two. Being a pastor, you know?"

"Of course," he responded, and thoughtfully pressed his palms together.

I took a deep breath and it all tumbled out of me, "The blizzard. Why the blizzard? Why a blizzard the weekend my dad died? A crippling blizzard at the worst possible time for my family. I'm having a lot of anguish over that. If you can't answer my question, it's fine. I guess I'm just looking for some theological insight."

Pastor Al smiled and crossed his arms. "Great question. I have a whole bunch of questions just like that one to ask when I arrive in heaven. My list of questions and I will be meeting God at the pearly gates. But it sounds as though you're looking for an answer now. It's one that I'm afraid I don't have, but I will tell you that sometimes when I'm searching for answers, I pray, and then I pray again. I talk with Kathy. I reach out to fellow clergy. And then I wait. The answers don't always come, but with time, I always find the strength to move on without one. You're about to bring your firstborn home; you've been blessed, Laura. Your son needs for you to move on."

I sat silent for a moment, thinking on his comforting words. And then I actually felt better. Like a ray of light had just peeked through a cloudy sky. He asked me if I wanted to pray with him. I said yes. At "Amen," I pushed the blankets aside and started to work my way out of bed.

Pastor Al held my arm to steady me and I asked, "Would you walk with me to the nursery to see Alex?"

"Of course," he replied. "As long as I have a chance to hold him."

When we left the hospital the next day, one of the nurses said to me, "Better pick up a six pack of beer on your way home with this one." Nothing I'd learned in college or life to that point could have prepared me for the challenge of bringing home a colicky baby.

The family labeled Alex a "screamer." I couldn't wait to return to work. His colic was so bad, he required medication to help him calm down and sleep. If he didn't take it, I would have needed it in very large doses. Little things would send him over the edge—airplanes flying overhead, a sudden movement, loud noises. I remember visiting Bill's stepmom and her husband with Alex in tow. He'd just fallen asleep in the bunting my mom had sewn for him.

I laid him gently on the bed, looked at Bill's family and out of sheer desperation and exhaustion said, "If anyone touches him and wakes him up, *you* will rock him and *you* will settle him down."

In the fall of 1988, my family was introduced to a medical geneticist from the University of Minnesota named Dr. Richards. Somehow, perhaps through one of my sisters, he'd heard there was a large family with FAP, all living in the Twin Cities. One evening in September, Dr. Richards and a registered nurse showed up to draw blood from us, right there in our mother's kitchen. The race to develop a genetic test was on, and Dr. Richards was in the mix of researchers hoping to discover the location of the genetic mutation that ran in our family. An accurate genetic test for FAP remained elusive. We all signed consent forms, but I couldn't participate because I was pregnant with our second child at the time. At almost thirty years old, I was continuing my exams with Dr. Schultz and remained polyp-free, but I was disappointed not to be part of Dr. Richards work.

Another thing I remember about that evening was a comment Dr. Richards made. He said something like, "If we can figure out familial polyposis, we might also be able to figure out sporadic colon cancers." I took that to mean people diagnosed without a family history of colon cancer. We knew we had a dominant gene in our family that equated to a virtual

100 percent chance of colon cancer in a carrier. Up to that point, we'd stayed on top of it with regular colon exams, postponing the inevitable colostomies for as long as possible. But it felt good to know that our blood donations might end up helping more people than just those in our family.

CHAPTER 11: **BENCH STRENGTH (1975-1986)**

Few would argue that the path to scientific discovery is easy.

In the 1970s, Dr. Cuthbert Dukes' laboratory assistant, HJR Bussey, years after being awarded a PhD for his work in polyposis, became world-famous for his knowledge about the condition. His thesis, "Familial Polyposis Coli. Family Studies, Histopathology, Differential Diagnosis, and Results of Treatment," published by Johns Hopkins Press in 1975, is considered a milestone in FAP literature.

In 1977, Frederick Sanger developed the classical "rapid DNA sequencing" technique, now known as the Sanger method, to determine the order of bases in a strand of DNA. Special enzymes are used to synthesize short pieces of DNA, which end when a selected "terminating" base is added to the stretch of DNA being synthesized. Typically, each of these terminating bases is tagged with a radioactive marker, so it can be identified. Then the DNA fragments, of varying lengths, are separated by how rapidly they move through a gel matrix when an electric field is applied—a technique called electrophoresis.

Frederick Sanger shared the 1980 Nobel Prize in Chemistry for his contributions to DNA-sequencing methods. The advent of even more advanced DNA-sequencing methods in the '80s would accelerate biological and medical research and discovery. In 1983, the polymerase chain reaction, or PCR, was invented. The PCR is used to amplify DNA. This method allowed researchers to quickly make billions of copies of a specific segment of DNA, enabling them to study it more easily. That same year, the first disease gene was mapped—a genetic marker for Huntington's disease was found on chromosome 4.

Fueled by a growing interest in cancer genes and more advanced laboratory techniques, researchers soon identified the faulty gene that was at the core of our polyposis condition. In 1986, a research team from the U.S. published a paper describing a man with FAP who was found to have a region missing from one of his two copies of chromosome 5. It would still be two years before Dr. Richards came to our house on Shryer Avenue to draw blood from my siblings as part of the effort to help locate the specific "address" of the gene mutation.

Later that same year, in October of 1986, the Minneapolis Star Tribune published an article from Newhouse News Service entitled, "Jaw, Eye May Give Clues to Colon Cancer Risk." Using studies dating back to the early 1970s, Johns Hopkins University researchers had discovered subtle changes to the jaw and eye that accurately predicted those who suffered inherited forms of colon cancer.

This was confirmation that Shelby's bony jaw tumor was related to her future diagnosis of FAP. In fact, both the jaw tumor and the shin cyst my nieces presented with as children were forewarnings of their inherited disease long before they were old enough to undergo colorectal screening and before the specific gene mutation was identified. We didn't know to make those connections because the work of researchers often takes years and was rarely published outside of academic institutions and professional journals.

Over time, I developed a much greater understanding of what my parents went through and wished I could take back my snide, "You polluted the gene pool" comment to my mother in 1979. Knowing how much those words must have hurt her breaks my heart to this day.

CHAPTER 12: **EBBS AND FLOWS**

When Alex's sister arrived in January of 1989, it seemed easier—almost like I'd earned the chance to experience a "normal" infant. Kelsey Evelyn was one of the most beautiful babies I'd ever seen. She was the biggest of our three children at birth—round face, light reddish-brown hair and amaranth-pink cheeks. Her eyes were a dark blue that over time became a gold-flecked green. I used to walk around Rosedale Mall with her while Alex was in preschool, and the other moms shopping there would often stop me and ask if they could take a closer look. Kelsey would oblige them with a sweet, shy smile and then turn and bury her face into her favorite blanket. Kelsey was colicky as well but only in the evenings—nothing that a warm bath and a little rocking couldn't cure.

When you have small children, you tend to find and gravitate to places that not only provide respite, but where your children are welcome as well. There was a small coffee shop in White Bear Lake called Coffee and Tea Ltd. that I'd often stop at with Alex and Kelsey securely strapped in the double stroller. I loved the woman behind the counter. She was much older than I was and a great storyteller. She made a wonderful café latte and shared with me that she was the mother of six, divorced, and now had grandchildren. Among her six kids were two sets of twins, born twelve months apart. I asked how she'd managed four infants so close in age.

Her reply has stayed with me all these years, "It was a blur. I don't remember how I managed, or even much about them at that age. It was really all about survival."

Bill became a divisional VP for American Express, which contributed greatly to my decision to leave Marsh and McLennan. I wanted to be busy but not so much so that the time with my own kids would become "a blur." It was to be a temporary change of plans. I remember my colleagues at Marsh sending me good wishes on the arrival of my daughter—"the perfect family" they would say.

I laughed and thought, *Just give me a few years to mess things up a bit.*

Those were wonderful days. I volunteered with several organizations while enjoying my time at home with our children. Apparently still not feeling busy enough, I used an experience I'd had with Kelsey as a crawling six-month-old to design an infant product called Kneetogs. I still remember stuffing little kneepads into plastic bags for shipping to distributors at 2:00 a.m. While my husband was impressed with this stroke of entrepreneurialism, I decided when my daughter Adele (Addy) Elisabeth arrived in December of 1992, that it was time to consider going back to school to work on obtaining my master's degree. I was concerned that I was growing less employable with each passing year out of the "real" workforce. The joy of Addy's arrival and her easy-going nature kept me from taking that leap back to school until she was a little older. It was as if she had slipped right into our busy lives and become the "van kid"—the one who winds up carted around town with Mom and Dad while we participated as a family in Alex and Kelsey's burgeoning school, social, and organized sports activities. It was so very different from the way I'd grown up as "free-ranger" in the neighborhood. And Addy had the best of attitudes. Van kid? No problem, she was just happy to come along for the ride. She was born with the most rose-colored of dispositions. As my neighbor Curt once said, "a quarter inch of new snow and that kid is out in the front yard on her sled."

My mother naturally evolved even more into the role of world's greatest grandmother after she was widowed. Without my dad or her own kids to take care of anymore, she continued to offer her home to others who needed a temporary place to stay, be it a grandchild, an old friend from the neighborhood, or the occasional rescue dog. Her grandkids were always on her mind; she adored being a grandmother. I'd stop at her house on my way home from something, and she'd immediately ask where the kids were. She was quick to offer her services as a live-in nanny for Bill and I when we were out of town. And my kids loved having her stay with them. She would bring Cookie Crisp cereal and a carton of real cream to pour over it for breakfast when she stayed overnight. She'd also bring craft supplies for Kelsey. Those two could concentrate for hours working on kid-friendly sewing and painting projects—activities I would have run screaming from as a little girl.

Another shared activity the two of them loved was coming up with ideas together for the costumes for Kelsey's plays. In the summer between kindergarten and first grade, she'd signed up for her elementary school's summer theater program. She'd caught the acting bug; I totally saw it coming...

I'd seen Phantom of the Opera at the Ordway Theater with my friend Jackie earlier in the spring. We both splurged on the soundtrack. I played it over and over again, singing along while I cleaned the house or played Legos with the kids. Over time, Kelsey came to know the story quite well—whenever I'd play the soundtrack she'd relentlessly ask me what was happening in the story. She often asked me to put in the tape while she ran to find Alex's black Dracula cape and a black Zorro mask that covered her eyes. She'd tuck a Kleenex under one side of the mask, attempting to look like the Phantom just before the beautiful Christine ripped off his mask. She never pretended to be Christine—she always preferred the Phantom. While the music played, she'd run around the living room in her mask and cape asking, "Now, Mom? Now? Do I pull the mask off now?" When I prompted her at just the right moment in the soundtrack, she'd yank her mask off, Kleenex and all, and give me her best diabolical laugh.

That love for the antagonist prepared her for roles as the Ugly Troll and the Big Bad Wolf in the two summer school plays the kids put on for their friends and families. I'm not sure what made my mom more proud as she sat in the audience— Kelsey bravely playing the lead roles in both productions or the perfect costume design she had visualized and sewn up on stage.

The early '90s were also a time of change for my brothers and sisters. Karen and Mark had moved to Texas with their family, and Debbie and Ron moved to Maryland with their two kids. For the first time, we were no longer all together in Minnesota.

The inherited familial polyposis syndrome continued to affect our family during this time as, one-by-one, a new generation closed in on adolescence. The recommended age for screening was still around thirteen—the age that I'd first met Dr. Schultz and his dreaded scope. My mother, in keeping with her consistent and frustrating non-compliance with doctors recommendations, had quit seeing Dr. Schultz altogether. Her reasoning was that as her colon had been totally removed, there was no reason to go—*how could one develop colon cancer without one?* I think she occasionally showed up for low hemoglobin and the occasional flu shot, but as a role model for staying on top of her health, to my mind she'd always been woefully deficient.

Marcie, Lisa, and I continued with colon screening every few years, even though most gastroenterologists would have said by then that, based on our histories and examinations, we weren't carriers of the mutated gene. As far as I was aware, there was still no accurate genetic test for familial adenomatous polyposis. It could be very frustrating—frustrating for those that knew they had it and now had to make sure their children received the same invasive screening, and for the three of us who didn't know for sure.

As had been the case in 1972, subtotal colectomies would be performed on the kids who presented with polyps. But a difference of opinion had developed among gastrointestinal doctors and colorectal surgeons in the intervening years. One side—quickly becoming the minority opinion—advocated for sticking with subtotal colectomies and regular screenings like my family had undergone. The other encouraged complete removal of the colon and rectum at the first sign of polyps, which would eliminate the need for the kind of aggressive surveillance my family had been subjected to. But that method, some doctors argued, might adversely impact the quality of life for patients who would undergo the procedure at such a young age. Even with new options that sometimes involved creating a bag or "pouch" inside the body—essentially eliminating the need for an external colostomy bag—there were still risks of absorption issues and whether or not there was enough healthy colon and small intestine to connect and create this pouch.

Members of the family moving to other states meant they'd be receiving advice and undergoing their surveillance procedures by different teams of doctors than we had here in Minnesota. The shifting tides of health insurance coverage and employment status didn't help matters, either. The advantages of us all seeing the same "family" doctor for a virtual lifetime had come to an abrupt end. Karen and her family started seeing doctors at MD Anderson in Texas. After moving to Maryland and learning their daughter, Andrea, had inherited the gene mutation that leads to FAP, Debbie and her husband selected Johns Hopkins in Baltimore. Fortunately, the hospital was already internationally recognized as a "center of excellence" for patients with the syndrome. In Minnesota, several of us continued to see Dr. Schultz because our health insurance companies allowed it, and we were comfortable with him. He knew our family and situation better than anyone.

What troubled me was that we were all being treated as individuals now, as opposed to a collective unit. I sensed that some of us might be receiving certain advice and recommendations that others weren't, and I found that unsettling. I was concerned that between the changes in insurance, different doctors, and not seeing or talking with each other as often, important information related to FAP might be missed and thus would not be shared among us. It was an uneasy feeling that subsided over time and was eventually buried beneath the commotion of our busy lives.

I remember Alex coming home with a creative writing assignment when he was in the fourth grade: "What job is the most important?" I was standing in the kitchen at the counter cleaning up after dinner and he asked, "How can a kid know what jobs are the most important if they've never had a job?" Despite having a grandmother who'd drive him to Wisconsin to buy illegal fireworks, he'd given up on the idea of working in a Chinese fireworks factory after learning that China was a long way from home.

Kelsey interjected that she thought the ladies who gave out food samples at the grocery store looked happy, so that must be a good job. I steered the conversation toward their studies in school. Kelsey was in first grade so most of her time was spent on the basics—reading, writing, arithmetic and getting along with others. And, of course, acting.

Alex, on the other hand, had been in school long enough to determine his "favorite" subjects outside of recess and gym. He'd come a long way from his first day of first grade—a full day of sitting in a classroom. He stumbled down those huge school bus steps and onto our driveway with three-year-old Kelsey running to him, her arms flung wide to greet him. He slammed his backpack on the ground, shot me a disgusted look, and pointed at me, saying, "Do you have any idea how long *six* hours is?"

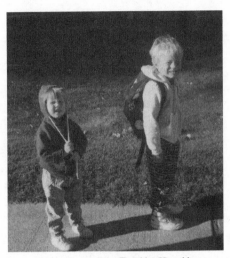

Alexander and the Terrible, Horrible,
No Good, Very Bad Six-Hour Day

Alex was a good reader but not bookish. I had to find books and magazines for him to read that kept his interest: *The World's Dumbest Criminals, Ripley's Believe It or Not,* the *Goosebumps* series, and the occasional *National Geographic Kids* magazine were his ideas of great reading material. I smiled, watching the pensive expression on his face while he contemplated the topic of his writing assignment. When prompted, he told me that he liked science best, then math. His over-the-top scientific curiosity was clearly evident, even as a toddler. I recall driving somewhere with him when he was about eighteen months old and quite the talker for his age. He constantly asked me questions, but one in particular stumped me. I honestly didn't know the answer. It was something silly like, "Laura (he called me Laura at that age and even pronounced the "L" correctly), "why are robin's eggs blue and duck eggs brown?" The science questions often baffled me, unfortunately. I searched around in my head trying to come up with something that would be satisfactory to him until I just looked at him sitting in his car seat through the rear-view mirror and said, "I don't know. I don't know the answer, Alex." He quickly excised the sippy cup from his mouth and announced with furrowed brows, "Then make something up!"

When he was two, Bill and I took Alex to the Science Museum of Minnesota to see the sarcophagus exhibit. I'd held him up to the glass to see the small Egyptian mummy and explained that it was a person who'd lived many thousands of years ago and that she'd been buried that way.

On the way home, a small voice came from behind me, "Laura?"

I turned to face him in his car seat. "Yes, Alex?"

"When I die, will they put me in a box?"

I whirled back to Bill and blurted, "Dad's taking us to Dairy Queen. Ice cream for everyone!"

A few days later he had typed up and printed off his answer to the question posed in his creative writing assignment. I found it lying on top of his backpack by the front door. It was only a paragraph long, but the words "Medical Researcher" jumped out at me:

I think a Medical Researcher has the most important job because if we didn't have them, we would have a lot of diseases going around and we wouldn't have any way to cure them. Medical researchers have helped cure some pretty nasty illnesses like polio, leprosy, smallpox, diphtheria and many more. In 1346, the plague known as Black Death struck Europe. If that happened today, Medical Researchers would probably find a cure for it before it hurt anyone. Medical researchers also help doctors. Medical research was the reason doctors could perform a successful human heart transplant. Today Medical Researchers are working on a cure for AIDS, cancer, heart disease, and unexplained hair loss (Ha, Ha). By Alex Kieger

Medical research, I thought. He must have been picking up on our family's conversations regarding the polyposis syndrome we'd inherited. It made me both proud and hopeful.

CHAPTER 13: **AUBURN-HAIRED GIRL**

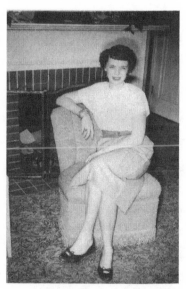

Our mother, circa 1953

The summer of 1997 was a hectic one. My nephew would be marrying in Illinois in August. Logistically, it presented the challenge of coordinating matching dresses and tuxedos for multiple members of the family living in different cities. My mom was busy at home putting the final touches on the fiancée's bridal gown as well as sewing dresses for the flower girls. She started the project in April with the intense fervor of a madwoman—this was her kind of event.

Before we took the trip to Illinois for the wedding, Bill and I celebrated our anniversary in Duluth. We stayed overnight at the local Radisson after seeing Collective Soul in concert at the convention center. I made a mental note to check in with my mom when we returned, as she'd declined to babysit while we were out of town celebrating because she wasn't feeling very well. That was worrisome, in and of itself, because she rarely passed up a chance to spend time with her grandkids. For a woman who'd had her colon removed twenty-five years earlier and rarely saw a doctor, she seemed to be in remarkably good general health. I made a point to tell her that I'd take her in right away when I returned if she wasn't feeling any better.

That was the week of July 20. That Sunday we were sitting in an urgent care waiting room at the same hospital where my father had passed away. There were urgent care locations closer to her home, but she insisted on Midway. It's funny how people continually gravitate to what's familiar. I remember my mother fretting about finding the newborn nursery at United Hospital when Alex was born. "Why couldn't you have your baby at a nice small hospital like Midway?" she'd asked.

So we sat in a room at Midway waiting for a medical provider to take a look at my mother. She was fatigued and had been for months. The frenzied sewing of wedding attire had masked how tired she really was. She had pain in her back. She looked jaundiced. Though I don't remember the exact details of that visit, the young woman who examined her—a physician's assistant I believe—merely suggested we set up an appointment for the following day with a primary care nurse practitioner. I asked her to draw some blood and run some tests. When she hesitated, my worry turned to anger. It was after 9:00 p.m., and we were both tired.

"Look at her," I said. "We're not leaving without some tests being done. If you don't do a blood draw and order tests, we'll leave and go to the emergency room at United Hospital."

Finally, the PA relented.

Mom's internal medicine doctors were the same that she and my dad had seen and trusted for years, so as far as I was concerned, we'd skip the nurse practitioner and go to the front of the line with the MDs.

When the results came back from the urgent care clinic, she was admitted upon her doctor's recommendation to St. Joseph's hospital in St. Paul. That would have been my mother's choice. Despite secretly attending confirmation and becoming a Lutheran, she never quit being fundamentally Catholic and St. Joe's—one of the first hospitals in Minnesota— had been founded by Catholic nuns. My mother just felt comfortable there.

The following Saturday we were hit with the devastating news. Eric and I were at my mom's house trying to corral one of her cats to bring to the Humane Society. I'd already found a home for her black lab with a family my neighbor knew. Despite all the stress and chaos of her illness, it was important to her that we made sure her pets were taken care of. While I was in between bolts of fabric in her basement trying to wrangle a cat from behind them, the phone rang. It was a doctor from the internal medicine practice. He'd been with the practice for years and knew both my dad and mom. He was sorry to break the news. My mother had advanced cancer in her liver—metastatic—most likely a primary cancer from somewhere else that had spread. He shared the findings with me over the phone while in the hospital room with my mother. They broke the news together. Stunned, I thanked him and, in a state of devastated shock, let Eric know.

The wedding was one week away.

The train is pulling out of the station, I thought, my head aching. *I've had this feeling before. It will start to pick up speed. It will move faster even though I'm trying to stop it. No matter what I do, nothing will change what's going to happen. I'll throw every ounce of my energy into controlling the situation. The illusion of control makes me feel strong when I am just an insignificant speck...*

Though my mother's prognosis was grave, she made it clear she wasn't interested in surgery or chemotherapy. She wanted to try "holistic" alternatives. We told her we would support any decisions she made around her care. Initially, our goal was to have Mom join us in Illinois. My cousin Joyce, a registered nurse, would accompany her and make sure she was comfortable on the plane and during the wedding. When we returned, Bill and I would rent a hospital bed and take my mother in so I could care for her as the disease progressed. It wasn't perfect, but at least it was a plan.

We talked a lot during those first frenzied days after she was admitted to St. Joe's, my mom and I. She seemed resigned to what was coming. She said she believed she'd been given more than one second chance to stay alive and raise her children—in 1957 when her colon polyps were first found and again in 1972 when she'd been diagnosed with colon cancer. She'd survived a genetic cancer predisposition syndrome that had taken her mother, her aunt, and her uncle in their thirties and felt she'd been given the additional years that they'd been deprived of. She said she never thought she would outlive my father and missed him terribly. She smiled and brought up our kids, making a point about how much she thought Kelsey was like her when she was a girl. "You know how we both love animals," she said, and I thought about how Kelsey would always pass up her dolls for her stuffed animals. Mom's eyes drifted to the window of her hospital room where a paper chain that Kelsey had made for her hung from the frame. "Please tell her how much her paper chain brightens up my room." I said I would.

During another of those early morning conversations, my mom mentioned that she'd had a visit from a catholic nun about their hospice program. The hospice was in a separate wing of the hospital and was known for providing excellent, compassionate end-of-life care. I asked my mother what she thought.

"I'm not sure," she said and suggested we talk more about it after the family meeting we'd scheduled with her doctors.

I made a point to be at the hospital for "doctor's rounds." An oncologist who'd seemed to arrive out of nowhere joined my mother's care team. He wasn't affiliated with St. Joe's but rather with a local private oncology practice. I don't recall exactly how he'd become involved because Mom had made it clear that she didn't want surgery or chemo and wanted to look at alternative options for everything from pain control to diet. But he was insistent. He suggested a biopsy of her liver so he could "better treat" her condition. When I asked him why this needed to be done, he accused me of "standing in the way of my mother's care." Yet even her internal medicine doctor, the one that broke the bad news to Eric and I the previous Saturday had suggested that everything be minimally invasive at that point. But my mom acquiesced. "Laura, don't argue with the doctor," she said.

He's not listening, I thought. *She's getting on a plane with an RN, and she's going to a family wedding in Illinois—you don't need to poke around her liver.* But with a quick nod of her head, my mother gave that oncologist the "go" to conduct the biopsy. Within forty-eight hours of that procedure, he would return to tell her "there was nothing he could do," and "it was possible she'd have a heart attack from elevated potassium levels." He then asked if she would prefer "going out that way." In front of me, as if I wasn't there, he used those very words.

Following the biopsy, her condition quickly deteriorated. The oncologist didn't even have the decency to be present for the family meeting at the hospital; he showed up prior to the agreed upon time and quickly left before the rest of us arrived. He was a poor excuse for a doctor in a patient-centered care facility and on top of that, a coward.

My mom signed papers to change the executor of her estate from Debbie to me, as Debbie was living in Baltimore at the time. Mom's signature was barely legible, her last attempt at signing her name to a legal document. Marcie was granted power of attorney for her health care decisions. Then, together, we talked about the hospice unit. While it would have put my own mind at ease, she struggled with the idea of hospice—she hadn't yet given up on attending her grandson's wedding. She wanted to be there with all of us. But because the wedding was fast approaching, and with her uneasiness about hospice care hanging over our conversations, we had to make decisions based on her staying in the oncology unit. She finally admitted that her condition would make travel difficult, and that it was best she not leave the hospital. *Small steps,* I had to remind myself. That and, *I am not in control.* The decisions weren't mine to make. Through clenched teeth and a shaky resolve to not start crying in front of her, I asked which of the kids she wanted to stay behind with her while we were in Illinois. She held up two fingers. Two of us would stay, the rest were to go and be present for my nephew and my sister. She didn't want anything to ruin the wedding. We weren't to tell Debbie how serious her condition was—"end stage, no heroics"—until after the reception.

I couldn't possibly go, I told her. It was all too much. Bill could drive the kids to Illinois and keep an eye on them without me. Again she held up two fingers.

Damn, I thought. *It's like she's sending us away.*

In the end, we decided that only Marcie, Butch, and Walt would stay behind. That way they could each take eight-hour shifts with her, never leaving her alone. Marcie's presence was imperative since she'd be directing my mother's care. My cousin Joyce would be with her as well. Everyone else was either taking part in the ceremony or had kids participating and would go to Illinois. Our plan was to make it through the wedding and then immediately after the reception, tell Debbie that she needed to grab the first flight to Minneapolis. In the meantime, I'd have to put on a poker face and lie if asked how Mom was doing. The lack of transparency nauseated me, but those were my dying mother's final wishes.

Just when you think the situation can't be more despairing, a light appears. This light came in the form of a housekeeper who came to my mom's hospital room with gloved hands and a rag for dusting, along with a few other items for tidying up her room. She wore a nametag that said "Maryann."

She was short and heavyset with brown hair, and had a constant smile on her face. She was a breath of fresh air compared to the oncologist. As she shuffled around the room, I mentioned our dilemma: that the majority of the family was leaving town for a wedding, and we were worried that my mother wouldn't receive the care she needed in the oncology unit.

Maryann was a big advocate of the hospice staff. She said they were caring and spiritual providers, and that my mother would be in good hands with them. She pulled the curtain closed on my mother's side of the double room and started up a conversation with my mom as she dusted the table near her bed, asking if she was comfortable. I could hear this from the other side of the curtain, but couldn't hear everything they talked about.

After about ten minutes, the curtain opened and Maryann walked past me and said, "She's ready to go now."

Not quite understanding what she meant, I didn't respond. I left the room to grab a cup of coffee in the hospital cafeteria and to make some calls to my siblings to update them.

When I returned, my mom looked up at me and said, "I think I want to go to the hospice unit."

It was the day before we were planning to leave to drive to Illinois for the rehearsal and the wedding. *Finally,* I thought, *something positive has happened.* It felt like a massive weight had been lifted off my shoulders.

In spite of what was going on behind the scenes—at least to those of us who knew what was happening back home—the wedding took place on a spectacular August day in 1997. I held it together as best I could until the processional. Addy wore a white dress with short-capped sleeves and a light gold sash around her waist and carried a spray of flowers alongside Eric's four-year-old daughter who wore a matching dress with her hair pulled into a high ponytail.

As the bridal party began their walk down the aisle, Bill whispered in my ear, "Your mom is making quite the entrance." I broke down then. He meant the dress, of course. It was beautiful, and everyone in attendance could see the finery and detail on the gown so lovingly sewn by my mom. I'm not sure what you call a heart that is both heavy and buoyant at the same time, but that is how I felt watching my nephew's wife-to-be walk gracefully down the aisle.

By the time the reception wound down and family pictures had been taken by the wedding photographer, word had made it back to Eric that Mom had passed away. As I left Eric's room and made the short, excruciating trip toward Debbie and Ron's room, I was racked with guilt. In my mind, I was thirteen again, reluctantly making my way to my mother's bedroom following her surgery. But this abrupt transition from joy to grief was much more devastating. So many of our final goodbyes went unspoken.

My mom died exactly one week from the day her doctor had called to tell Eric and I she had metastatic cancer. As painful as it was, it didn't come as a surprise to me. I'd sensed when I left the hospital that last time I wouldn't see her again, and that thought had stayed with me the entire time we were in Illinois.

But I knew, on the other side, my father would be waiting for her. The auburn-haired girl from North Dakota who'd married him in 1947 was with him once again. And that's how things were supposed to be.

When we were kids, my mother told us that when she died, we should donate her body "to science." She wanted doctors to learn more about familial polyposis and what it had done to her family, and perhaps discover something that would someday help her children and grandchildren. We never took that directive seriously. Not only did we fail to donate her body to science, we didn't have an autopsy done either. We never talked about it. Her cancer had started somewhere and then metastasized to her liver. Where did it start? We weren't given the time to find out.

After the funeral—at which there were no lilies—I threw myself into the role of executor of what was left of my parents' estate. Selling the house on Shryer Street—the house my dad and his brothers and my grandfather built—was agonizing. It was all so *final*. After that, it was dividing up what was left between the eight kids. My responsibilities meant that I had to take a break from graduate school. At that point, the only thing I had left to do before I finished was a final paper and presentation to faculty. But that would have to wait. I had more important issues to focus on.

About a month after my mother's death, I stopped at Target to pick up a "thank you" card to drop off at St. Joseph's. I was feeling especially grateful that she'd passed away in the hospice unit surrounded by such caring individuals who'd also helped my sister and two brothers through what had been a very difficult time. Before I left for St. Joseph's, however, I called down to the hospital to make sure I knew where I was going and to be sure I had the spelling of Maryann's name right for the card. I wasn't sure what her last name was because it hadn't been on her nametag. I just knew her as Maryann. I called down to the hospice unit—no luck. I asked to be transferred to housekeeping—no Maryann that they knew of. They put me on hold as they asked around. Then I called the oncology floor and described her in detail. They couldn't help me. They had no record of a Maryann *ever* working in housekeeping. I thought perhaps she'd been fired or quit. Maybe she'd been from a temp agency. Puzzled and a bit frustrated, I gave up on the idea of leaving her the "thank you" card and ended the call.

The night of the wedding, the photographer took a family picture at the reception. We all look so happy—Bill, so handsome in his suit, Alex with his fresh haircut and navy polo, Addy in her gorgeous flower girl dress, and Kelsey wearing an adorable straw hat adorned with pink fabric roses and green petals that she must have picked out herself. So odd that it was taken right around the time my mother drew her last breath. To this day, it is one of my favorite pictures of the five of us together.

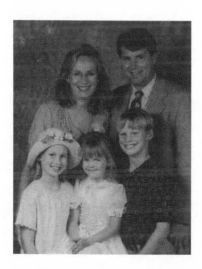

CHAPTER 14: FINALLY, A TEST

The year following my mother's death, 1998, was marked by a series of musts—must settle the estate, must finish my final paper for grad school, must look for a new job in human resources. It was time. With a combination of preparation and a little luck, I was hired as the Human Resources Director at a community hospital just east of the Twin Cities. In spite of the eighty-mile round-trip commute, I loved working with healthcare professionals whose commitment to patients was apparent every day.

My brother Eric wasn't far behind me on the job change trajectory. True to what we'd always expected, he'd become a cop and had worked as a police officer for years in the community. He was mulling over the idea of applying for a promotion to sergeant within the department. It would be an important step in his career, but he was concerned he wouldn't be able to continue working with his canine partner, Cooper. Cooper had become part of the family. Eric used to proudly show off pictures of his "bites"—most of them, I teased, looked to be from the calves of petty shoplifters fleeing the local shopping mall.

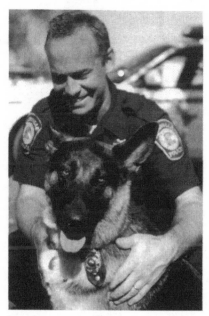

Eric and his K9 partner, Cooper

When Eric and his family went on vacation, Bill was tasked with the care and feeding of Cooper. He took it very seriously, precisely measuring out his food and making sure not to use certain words and phrases around him—commands that Eric only used when Cooper was on duty. I guess Eric didn't trust me; I was too talkative, and his gentle ribbing of me about my driving record suggested he had the absurd impression that I was easily distracted.

Funny, because I often teased him when he was behind the wheel. On more than one occasion I told him, "Not all road trips need to replicate high-speed chases, you know?"

He'd laugh and say, "It's a cop thing."

"And what does that mean?" I asked.

"Well Sis," he said, with a sage look and a droll grin, "I am the recipient of many hours of advanced skills training in defensive driving and super cool maneuvers behind the wheel. You, on the other hand, are the recipient of numerous traffic citations. But the department thanks you for your many contributions to our revenue stream."

I gave him a playful slug on the shoulder. That was the other fun thing about Eric—like my dad, he had a terrific sense of humor.

Helping Eric update his resume and draft a cover letter in preparation for applying for the sergeant's job was one of those great sibling bonding experiences. He would face multiple interviews and assessments as part of the advancement process. I literally had to pull the self-promotion out of him. He'd never been much of a braggart. He was fortunate to have inherited the best of my parents—my dad's courage, humility, conscientiousness, and good humor, along with my mom's love of animals and sense of responsibility for others. Even as a kid, he possessed natural leadership traits—he kept his commitments and always acted with integrity, even fessing up when he got into trouble. People naturally gravitated to him— why was it so hard for him to put that into words? As he sat next to me in uniform while I typed, I couldn't help but believe he'd nail the interviews and convince the search committee that he was the best candidate to become their newest sergeant. Not to mention, he had those super cool driving skills.

At that time, I was fast approaching forty and my regular exams with Dr. Schultz continued to show me free of polyps. Patients around the world struggling with familial cancer syndromes were benefitting from major advancements in the understanding of genetics and human disease that had occurred within the previous ten years.

The discovery of the APC gene in 1991 and the understanding of how it "worked" was a watershed moment for scientists and geneticists studying FAP. Dr. Schultz suggested I have the screening done in order to confirm that I was not a carrier, and I could then start to have colonoscopies like normal people—every five years or so. Dr. Schultz was also nearing retirement, and the thought of starting up with a new doctor was not something I looked forward to—especially after having one who knew our family and history so well.

Dr. Schultz's goal had been to keep our colons healthy for as long as he could. He wanted us to have quality of life—to be able to fall in love, marry, have families, and hopefully grow old without the potentially life-altering problems and complications associated with removing the colon before it became necessary. I wasn't entirely sure who to see once Dr. Schultz retired or what to expect from a new colorectal surgeon or gastroenterologist, who—even within their own specialties—had wide divergences of opinion on how best to treat those with FAP. Surveillance, surgery, and/or involvement in clinical trials of new drugs to help reduce the numbers of polyps—the opinions were many and varied and the options growing, which sometimes led to more confusion for us.

While we were relatively sure by then that I wasn't a carrier, there were still several considerations to think about before going through with the genetic test. On the plus side was the reassurance and reduction of anxiety about my hereditary cancer risk. I'd be able to avoid unnecessary procedures and potential surgeries. Perhaps most important would be the relief of knowing my own children were free from the increased risk. But on the other side of the coin, I'd run the risk of becoming complacent about the routine surveillance still necessary to protect me from problems that would otherwise be found by my advanced level of screening. And there was survivor's guilt and the potential for strained relationships with others in the family. In terms of the latter, there'd always been an understanding between the siblings as to which of us likely carried the gene mutation and to my recollection, there had never been any resentment or arguments about it. If there were any hard feelings at all, it was our frustration with my mother's stubborn refusal to go in for regular checkups when she knew full well that she was afflicted with the familial polyposis syndrome.

Ultimately, I took Dr. Schultz's advice and set up an appointment at the University of Minnesota to have the genetic test done.

It was required that I consult with a genetic counselor both at the time of the blood draw and the follow-up appointment at which I would receive my results, regardless of the findings. While there was a growing understanding of the psychological impact that inherited pre-dispositions to cancer might have on affected families, genetic-disease related family counseling was largely non-existent and primarily found in academic settings in 1972, when we could have used it the most. While Dr. Schultz did his best to offer advice and counsel, we were left to figure out the details on our own and had to learn to deal with the emotional fallout from our vicious and abrupt initiation to FAP and its consequences. It wasn't until the 1980s that the field of genetic counseling began to grow rapidly. With an estimated fifty million Americans having genetic conditions and some 5,000 diseases having been identified as being genetic in origin, the demand for services continued to expand.

My siblings were all doing okay—as long as they maintained their surveillance protocol and the doctors were able to burn, snare, or remove any suspicious looking polyps, they could live a relatively normal life, albeit with the knowledge that they may someday require a colostomy. That seemed a reasonable risk, given that our mother had lived to the age of sixty-seven despite her battle with FAP and the resulting surgeries.

What I knew going into the test was that FAP is caused by an alteration in the APC gene on chromosome 5, and that the mutation is inherited in an autosomal dominant manner as I'd learned in my college biology class listening to the lecture on inherited disease. Only one copy of the altered gene was necessary for symptoms of the condition to be present. In the simplest of terms, because my mother had FAP, the odds were fifty-fifty that her children would have inherited the mutated gene.

The APC gene mutation that leads to FAP accounts for approximately 1 percent of colon cancers worldwide. Interestingly, 20-25 percent of patients diagnosed with FAP are what the medical community calls "de novo" or "new," meaning that the mutation could not be traced back to a family member and had occurred spontaneously in the patient. Doctors also refer to these as "isolated cases." And just like those who'd inherited the disease, a "de novo" familial polyposis patient will also have a fifty-fifty chance of passing on the condition to their offspring.

As difficult as it is to accept that one might have inherited an autosomal dominant syndrome like FAP, the thought of this syndrome occurring "de novo" seemed especially cruel. These cases are often diagnosed in young adults—twenty-five or thirty-year-olds finding out for the first time that their gastrointestinal tract is peppered with polyps, or worse. Our situation could hardly be described as a picnic, but at least we all knew what to watch for and had a chance to catch potential problems early.

I arrived at the University clinic to receive my results. As required, the genetic counselor was there with me. The lab slip read, "Familial Adenomatous Polyposis—Unknown Mutation." The result was somewhat confusing, but at least I had more information moving forward:

Result: Negative for segments 1-5. (No truncated protein identified.) This does not rule out FAP.
Comment: This assay can identify about 80% of the mutations causing FAP. This test cannot identify mutations that do not cause protein truncation abnormalities. Therefore, 20% of people affected with FAP will have a negative result. Other types of familial colorectal cancer are not detected by this test. Diagnosis of FAP should not rely on molecular testing alone, but should take into consideration clinical symptoms.

The genetic counselor was a friendly and soft-spoken woman who wore glasses perched on the end of her nose. I didn't know exactly how to process the information she shared with me, but I took the test results to be largely positive. I thanked her for her time and left the University feeling like the dots were starting to connect. My early "clean" diagnosis based solely on clinical presentation—the many years of colon exams with no evident polyps—now synced up with a genetic test with an 80 percent accuracy rate. In my mind, it was enough to finally convince myself that I'd not inherited the APC mutation that could lead to colorectal cancer.

As I began my walk to the parking ramp, I stopped to sit on an empty bench in front of a small campus church bathed in bright summer sunlight. Students rushing to their next classes passed by. I recognized myself in them. A student sitting in a class called Heredity and Human Society in 1979—on this very campus—seeing my life represented by an as yet unshaded circle on a pedigree chart of FAP carriers in my family. Perhaps they wondered, *What is that woman thinking?* If they could have peered inside my head, they would have seen a thousand difficult moments flashing behind my eyes. But this moment was a good one, filled with relief and gratitude.

The intersection of the test results and the consult with the genetics counselor brought me back to my first year of graduate school—my first class, actually. It was developmental psychology, and I loved it. In that classroom, I learned that the yellow blanket that Addy had carried around with her at all times when she was little and the laminated copy of my father's obituary that I kept in my wallet were known as transitional objects—reminders of special people and connections that were important to us.

As parents of three young kids, my old human development textbook sometimes still came in handy for Bill and me. In it was a quote about middle age that had been branded into my consciousness. Though I don't remember it exactly, it went something like, "When you are young, you look at your life in terms of *how much time you have in front of you*. But by middle age, that same mental orientation makes a dramatic shift and you then see your life *as the time you have left*."

In the end, your time is your life. Whenever you speak or think the word "time," replace it with the word "life."

It struck me at that moment, just how much of my time, my *life*, was dedicated to, well, busyness—the twin devils of distraction and preoccupation that "serves the same psychological role that it always has: to keep us sufficiently distracted that we don't have to ask ourselves potentially terrifying questions about how we are spending our days."

I needed to let certain tasks go undone, to say "no" more often. To be willing to sacrifice "stuff" for experiences. To invest in creating memories, not clutter. Travel. Volunteer. Be present. Essentially, I needed to do the things I loved most with the people I loved most. It was time to start planning.

CHAPTER 15: **TRULY LIVED MOMENTS**

I remember the first time Marcie convinced Debbie and me to go with her to Vail, Colorado. I'd never been skiing "out West." Standing at the top of Avanti run on the mountain, looking out over a panorama of snow and mountains and blue sky... It was a religious experience. When I closed my eyes I was thirteen again, marching down Dale Street, Kastle's on my shoulder, headed to mount Villa.

In 1999 we took a big family trip to Disneyworld with Debbie, Marcie, Walt, Lisa, Eric, and their families. We were bumped from our flight home due to overbooking and all of the inconvenienced travelers were given free round-trip airline tickets to fly anywhere in the US for our trouble. We picked Seattle—just because. We'd never been there, and it looked like a great city to visit. Between hiking around Mount Rainer and visiting the Space Needle and Pike Street Fish Market, we fit Seattle and Seattle fit us. Kelsey and Addy even caught a fish tossed to them by one of the "fish guys" at the Market. After a quick photo, they were anxious to give it back.

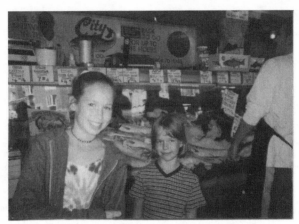

Kelsey and Addy at the Seattle Fish Market

In June of 2001, Debbie, Marcie, Lisa, and I along with Debbie's kids traveled to Paris. We stayed at the Hotel Latin located right in the heart of the Latin Quarter in the 5th arrondissement. The area was bustling with students and a trove of Parisian history.

It was my first trip to Europe. Debbie and Marcie had been to France several times, and both spoke French well. As long as Lisa and I didn't venture too far on our own, navigating the city would be a piece of cake. But after a few days in the City of Lights, my wanderlust set in. I love the feeling of being in a yet-to-be-explored city. You can leave your troubles behind for a while and reconnect with yourself. Immersing oneself into a completely different culture as a traveler of one can be incredibly restorative. Traveling with sisters, however, tends to be a group endeavor, but I eventually convinced them that I'd be fine exploring Paris on my own. I strolled the Left Bank of the Seine, retracing some of the steps I'd taken with my sisters and my niece Andrea on previous walks, past the Sorbonne and the Pantheon, passing student drinking holes and elegant café terraces. I sat down near the statue of St. Michael, a popular meeting spot for locals and tourists alike. I people watched for a bit, fascinated—young Parisians sitting at a bistro having a coffee with their hands intertwined across the table, enamored foreigners, their eyes wide with awe, shopkeepers waving potential customers into their stores. I overheard conversations in a language I didn't understand, but that sounded so beautiful. If I had but one word to describe Paris, it would be "captivating."

It was clear from the start how Andrea wanted to spend her time. Hanging out with your aunts was reserved for the day hours. She and her friend had other plans once the Parisian club scene started heating up around midnight. On those occasions we were graced with her presence, we caught up on her life in Baltimore. She told us about her job as an activities and marketing coordinator at the assisted living center, and her new boyfriend Johnny, who happened to be in a local rock band when he wasn't working for his family's business. We could tell she was crazy about him—she positively beamed anytime his name came up.

The trans-Atlantic flight back to the States from France gave me time to think about how different vacations had been for all of us growing up—especially how those trips out West with our parents compared to our children's travel experiences. My parents drove, of course, as it was cost prohibitive to fly with such a large family. But those road trips provided something more—the wonder of exploring the country in an entirely different way. My dad would point at the sky and ask, "What type of cloud is that?" I would run the names through my head—altocumulus, altostratus, stratus, cumulus, and stratocumulus. I rarely got it right. It was science, after all. But we saw the country. Not from 35,000 feet, but from behind the windows of a woodgrain-paneled station wagon. I remember the thrill of helping set up our camper at a KOA camp, and once released, running around looking for kids my age—boys or girls, it didn't matter. We'd exchange addresses and be pen pals for a while, then school would start up in the fall and the exchange of letters would become more and more infrequent. Then one day you come across them again while sifting through a box of souvenirs you barely remember collecting.

I saw the Pacific Ocean for the first time when I was nine or ten, amid long treks of the Midwestern plains and trips through mountain ranges like the Rockies and Tetons. We'd camped in Yosemite, Yellowstone, and Glacier National Parks in the U.S., and—when Lisa, Eric, and I became true road warriors—Banff and Jasper in Canada. The first time I saw the Grand Canyon as a fourteen-year-old, I had the same feeling that I would have standing on Vail Mountain almost thirty years later. I'd never imagined anything in the natural world could be so beautiful.

I wanted our kids to have those same kinds of experiences as well.

Our first interstate Kieger family road trip was in the summer of 2002. The plan was to drive to Iowa in two vehicles and hop an Amtrak bound for Denver. From there, we'd rent an SUV and drive to Telluride, Colorado, then on to the Grand Canyon, up through western Colorado, and then return to Denver where we'd take the train back to Iowa.

The second vehicle was for me—I had an extra leg of the trip planned. I'd take the Amtrak to Salt Lake City from Denver.

My friend Sarah would pick me up and we'd spend time together in Jackson Hole while Bill and the kids went back to Minneapolis. Two and a half weeks of vacation—I *almost* felt guilty.

As we drove through the San Juan mountain range and came into Telluride, a voice in the backseat said, "I didn't know towns like this existed." I don't remember which of the kids said it, but it warmed my heart because it was exactly what I was hoping to hear. *Just wait until they see the Grand Canyon,* I thought.

Ten days later I was on my way to Jackson Hole in Sarah's truck, excited to see her parents and to meet her sister's two children. Sarah had recently sold her house on the central coast of California and split her time between Tucson and Jackson Hole where she focused solely on her painting career—her work had been displayed in several major galleries in California and the southwest. She and a few of her artist friends were staying with another successful artist at his massive log home near the Snake River. His triple garage had been converted into a studio for other artists to use—potters, weavers, and painters alike. I met several of them while visiting and was asked to join them on a hike in the Tetons to look for huckleberries—which they claimed were great on pancakes—and elk antlers for one of the artists who used them as handles for woven baskets. I doubt my presence was all that helpful, but it was nice to be invited to tag along. It was well past 5:00 p.m. when our hiking, antler-hunting, and berry-picking came to an end.

I was anxious and watching the time, because I wanted to talk to Debbie in Baltimore where it was after 8:00. We were picking up a conversation regarding a strange call Andrea had received from her bank. The staff had noticed that her signature had changed, and they wanted to make sure no one was trying to forge her checks. She'd also started having trouble tying her shoes, and instead of asking herself why that might be, she just ran out and bought a couple pairs of slip-ons and tennis shoes with Velcro straps. During that phone conversation with Debbie, she mentioned Andrea's doctors had spotted small lesions on Andrea's brain, which were the likely culprits behind her compromised fine motor skills. They planned to monitor them for any changes.

Our second road adventure (also known as "too much family time" according to fourteen-year-old Kelsey) was the following summer. At that point extended vacations were easier to plan, as both Bill and I were self-employed. We decided to head east this time, traveling via a large passenger van complete with a DVD player for the kids, through Chicago and into Indiana. From there we traveled through Ohio and Pennsylvania, spending the night in Pittsburgh at a Super 8. Kelsey, unimpressed with the accommodations, asked upon learning we'd have to buy shampoo and conditioner for her shower from a vending machine, "How many stars is this place, anyway?" From Pittsburgh we headed southeast toward Maryland. We had a side trip planned but hadn't told our kids yet. That would be a surprise.

We arrived at Debbie and Ron's in Elkridge, Maryland road-weary but excited to eat Chesapeake Bay blue crabs soaked in Old Bay and to celebrate Andrea and Johnny's recent engagement. Andrea had made a full recovery from her previous shoelace tying and writing problems, and they planned to marry in June of 2005. Fortunately, their long, two-year engagement would give the families time to pull everyone and everything together.

The surprise was a three-day weekend in New York City. With Debbie in tow, we drove to Edison, New Jersey, parked the van, and took the train into Manhattan. We stayed in Herald Square at a boutique hotel frequented by international travelers. While I liked the global flair of the place, Kelsey overheard the desk clerk's conversation and whispered to me with a concerned tone and look of disgust on her face, "they rent rooms by the hour." I, of course, was mortified that my precocious fourteen-year-old daughter even knew what that might mean. But, it was in a great location with easy access to the subway system and was perfect for taking in the city. We were only there for a few days and had to maximize our time. Bill and Alex checked out the Intrepid, ESPN Zone, and the Hard Rock Café. The girls window-shopped in the garment district, checking out material and lace for bridal gowns. We found a quaint boutique fabric shop and quickly stepped in and began to examine the bolts of fabric and lace trim. The adept sewing and dressmaking skills of my mom and my older sisters had somehow completely missed me. For them it was a form of creative expression. It didn't help that in eighth grade sewing class, my final project was a simple halter-top that my mom had to help me complete in order to avoid an F. Like algebra, I saw no future need for these skills. I could, however, nail "couture" in a spelling bee.

Kelsey and Addy were intrigued as Debbie skillfully described the differences between the types of lace and why some was of higher quality than others. My girls listened intently. As she explained it (and in a way that their Grandma Colleen would have completely understood) "there's lace, then there's *real lace.*" I smiled at my sister, thinking about Mom and the beads she'd insisted be sewn on my own bridal gown.

I knew it was close to lunchtime when Addy, out of nowhere, burst out asking, "Can we eat sushi again under the skyscraper." We all laughed, and I suggested we try one of the local delis—her lunch, I promised, would be delicious and likely come with the best pickle that she'd ever tasted. We left the boutique in search of a classic, New York delicatessen and didn't have to travel very far. After our leisurely, pickle-fueled lunch we went to find Bill and Alex. We ended up together at Rockefeller Plaza and NBC studios and bought tickets to see the Saturday Night Live set.

At the close of our whirlwind adventure into NYC, we arrived at Grand Central Station and Debbie boarded a train back to Baltimore. Bill and I and the kids took the train to Edison, New Jersey to pick up our van and head home. The goal I'd set back in 2001 while flying over the Atlantic had been accomplished. Our kids had seen the country—the west, the east, and several states in between.

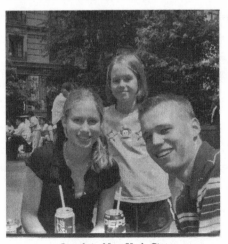

Lunch in New York City

By 2004, Andrea's wedding planning was in high gear, and she'd been promoted to Director at the assisted living facility where she was employed. She was busy working and saving up to buy a townhome not too far from her parent's house. I jumped at an opportunity to go to Washington D.C. late in the spring for a medical device and biotechnology conference in the hopes of spending some time in Baltimore with Andrea. It was nice to see her whenever I could. She'd left Minnesota when she was about fourteen, and I always worried she'd be so busy we would never see her—she didn't come back "home" much.

Every now and then, Bill and I would have a good laugh about the time Andrea was babysitting our son, and a bat came flying through the family room in the dead of winter. She took just enough time to bundle Alex up and then fled the house to take refuge at the neighbors, forgetting her own coat and shoes in the process. Her cousins loved her—she was fun and pretty and full of life and energy. And now she was engaged.

Andrea picked me up from the conference center in D.C. Before we went to Debbie and Ron's, we took a detour to her work. Andrea showed me her office and introduced me to her colleagues, but I sensed those were cursory introductions and she was more excited for me to meet the residents. They called her "Miss Andrea," and she beamed. She knew them all by first name along with their personal histories—where they'd worked and lived, their children and grandchildren. And of course she wanted to know how their days were going and if they'd gone to play bingo or down to the music room to listen to Miss Daisy play ragtime tunes for her fellow residents. I'd honestly never seen that side of her. She embraced those senior citizens like they were part of her family, and they responded with deep affection for her. As we walked back to her car I made a point to tell her how proud I was of her and what a great role model she had been to my girls. Before I disintegrated into a teary-eyed mess, I directed the conversation toward the wedding, and she ran with it the rest of the drive.

That trip to D.C. was a bit too short for my liking, but I needed to get back home to start planning for Alex's high school graduation in June. It's a custom in Minnesota to have a garishly huge graduation party. In any event, Midwestern tradition (and peer pressure) ensured we would be throwing a big bash for him as well. Mailing invitations, cleaning up the yard and garage, and attending the official graduation ceremony was all part of the process. Graduation, of course follows prom—what my friends refer to as "mini weddings"—which is preceded by Spring Break. We discovered that being the parents of a high school senior could be exhausting. And expensive.

Following graduation Alex went off to Drake University in Des Moines, Iowa. It pretty much met his criteria—a small-to-mid-sized regional university with a good reputation and "normal kids." (I wasn't entirely sure what he meant by that.) While he liked the feel of the University of Minnesota, he felt it was too big and too close to home. Though he'd started out declaring a biology major, an observant faculty member with the Biochemistry Department at Drake made a point of talking with him about career opportunities in the field, leading him to change his major before he'd even set foot on campus. He told us that professor's interest in him is what swayed his decision. *Good for him*, I thought. When I was in high school—destined for my future liberal arts degree—I'd needed to rely on nice, nerdy boys just to help me navigate applied chemistry. Bill and

I never could quite figure out where Alex had gotten his aptitude for math and science.

CHAPTER 16: **DIAGNOSIS**

In August of 2004 Eric turned forty, and we celebrated with a big deck party at his house. It was hard to believe Jerry and Colleen's youngest child was now forty years old, a highly respected and decorated sergeant with the police department. His birthday party brought my thoughts back to earlier summers when Eric volunteered for the Police Explorers program, getting used to dealing with the public while directing Minnesota State Fair traffic. He must have been in high school at the time. I'd drive through the congestion and watch him working, careful not to catch his eye and distract him from his duties. It seemed like such a big job for such a young man. But for him, directing traffic was just a warm-up. His attachment to the community in which he grew up is what drove his passion for the job and continued to fuel his successful career. We were so proud of him.

The summer of 2004 gave way to the summer of 2005. Between planning for Andrea's wedding, the trip to Baltimore, and preparing to see Alex off to college, the year passed in an apparent instant. It didn't help that the older I got the more fleeting the passage of time seemed.

Andrea and Johnny's wedding that June was everything she'd hoped it would be. Her cousins were part of the bridal party. The reception site was beautiful—a charming atrium converted from a 19th century working mill. And it provided an opportunity to have the whole family together again.

Looking back at the pictures from those three family gatherings—Alex's graduation, Eric's birthday party, and Andrea's wedding—they were celebrations I remember as some of the last that we felt completely happy and unencumbered by the kinds of health issues that had plagued our parents at those ages. We were all into our forties and fifties, on the cusp of enjoying our lives with our adolescent and adult children.

But late that fall, just after Thanksgiving, Eric started to complain of stomach pain. Initially, he'd not thought much of it, especially since the occasional antacid would sometimes help. He came to me and asked about my experience with gallstones and what they'd felt like before I had my gallbladder removed. I pointed to the hollow where my stomach met my ribs and said, "Excruciating pain. Right here." He told me his pain came and went and was never constant. I told him that he should go see the doctor and that there was no reason to be in pain if the antacids weren't working for him.

He went to see his gastroenterologist after Christmas and the doctor performed some kind of imaging workup. I don't recall what they were concerned about specifically at that time, but I vividly remember the subsequent phone call that I received from Marcie while sitting at my desk. His doctor had found some small lesions on Eric's liver, and it looked serious.

I practically knocked Mary Kay over on my way to the elevators. She walked in behind me and the doors slipped closed. She was a Masters prepared RN and our Director of

Clinical Research so she understood everything that came tumbling out of my mouth on the ride to the ground floor. As I exited I heard her say "and let me know if your family wants information on clinical trials—I can put you in touch with knowledgeable people who can help." I turned to look back at her and mouthed "thank you," before the elevator whisked her away.

I went straight to Eric's house, not bothering to stop at home. He was worried. We were all worried. I told him we were going to fight whatever it was, trying to stay strong for him, but secretly, inside, I was crumbling.

He was scheduled for a PET scan later that week to determine the stage of his disease and where the primary cancer might have originated. The results were devastating. Eric had an aggressive stomach cancer that had spread to his liver. By that time I could focus on nothing but his battle. And I was angry. I couldn't believe that it was happening—*again*—to another young family member. But even worse than the anger was the feeling I was failing him all over again, as I had in Anaheim when I neglected to catch him coming down the pool slide.

CHAPTER 17: BELOVED BROTHER

When someone you love is diagnosed with a serious illness, isolation casts a shadow over the fear. People are well intentioned. They ask, "How are things going?" and you respond with just enough information to keep them from inquiring further, because you don't want to break down at work or while shopping at the grocery store.

The fight to save Eric became the whole family's battle. The isolation and loneliness inherent in our fight could only be fathomed, felt, and unbridled with one another. The nephew who responds to an e-mail in the middle of the night, because he's lying awake running the same scenarios through his mind and worrying about what might come next. The sister who makes the two-hour drive down to Mayo Clinic, records in hand, trying to find a gastric cancer expert with an open calendar who might provide a second opinion and a chance at a hopeful outcome. And as much as we might have wanted to, we couldn't put our lives on hold—we had kids to raise, teenagers to keep an eye on, and work that had to be done in order to pay our mortgages and keep food in our refrigerators. Like any family that has experienced a serious medical situation, the constant din of daily life can't be muted. We're never alone, of course—friends and co-workers step in to share the anxieties and help us stay positive. But at the end of the day, it's just us, standing alone in the path of what comes next.

One night after my teenage daughters went to bed and soon after we learned of Eric's diagnosis, I went down into our basement where we kept our desktop computer. I wasn't sure where to start so I typed, "stomach cancer" into the search bar. I was hoping to find the best treatment options, clinical trials— anything out there that might help Eric. Back in the day of AOL's instant messenger service, my nephew and I would both be online late at night. While I scoured the Internet doing research, he had conversations with doctors in his home state. The two of us exchanged the information we'd found and discussed what some of the experts in the field had shared on the Web, sometimes until 2:00 a.m. Before blogs became popular, it was mostly white papers and technical research coming out of different cancer centers.

Based on what we found, none of the risk factors applied to Eric. Despite our family's predisposition to colon cancer, as far as we were aware, none of our relatives had ever been diagnosed with stomach cancer. He was young. He didn't smoke. And he was in great physical condition.

In between the many articles and abstracts, I also searched "how to make an appointment at Memorial Sloan Kettering" in New York and "how a physician can make a referral to MD Anderson" in Texas. My hope was to find Eric the best care in the country. What kept me going was the knowledge that my brothers and sisters were all doing the same thing. They too were up until all hours on their computers trying to figure things out.

Diagnosed at an advanced stage, as Eric's cancer was, the recommendation was to look for clinical trials. That pursuit required considerable time and Internet searches, but my energy never waned. I burned through ink cartridges and printer paper and hours, cobbling together a veritable arsenal of information.

But Eric remained the real hero. Out of concern for his family and his team of officers, he chose to be treated close to home. I'd heard that he'd sometimes show up to sign a search warrant dragging his chemo pump behind him. He arranged for a wireless laptop so that he could review and assign cases while undergoing treatment. He also continued his work to establish a police canine officer's health and wellness program in conjunction with the Veterinary Medical Center at the University of Minnesota. He checked his work e-mail and voicemail during hospitalizations. He truly loved his job and continued to serve the community with passion and dedication despite his pain and treatments throughout the spring and summer of 2006.

The last thing Eric wanted was to leave his job in order to focus on his illness full time, but eventually the choice was taken from him. Though his first round of chemo had successfully shrunk the tumors and lesions, his cancer roared back by fall.

Debbie's son and his family traveled to Minnesota to celebrate Thanksgiving with us. Those who could make it did, because no one was sure how much time Eric had left. No one imagined it would be mere days.

My beloved brother died that very Sunday—the Sunday of Thanksgiving weekend—with his family and fellow officers at his side until the end. None of us had even talked about a funeral—doing so would have meant giving up hope.

One of Eric's friends and colleagues provided a window into our broken hearts: "As you all know, I loved Eric for who he was. Eric was the toughest, but kindest person I have ever known. Always the pillar of support and care for all he knew. Eric earned the respect of his friends and co-workers because he was willing to stand up and fight for those things he thought were right. Eric rarely settled for the word 'no.' Always lending a helping hand whether I needed it or not, never once expecting anything from me in return. Eric taught me many things since we have known each other, but it was the last lesson I will always try to reflect upon; don't let the uncertainties of life keep you from living it. I will miss my dear friend. Until we meet again."

On the way to the cemetery, the roads were lined with saluting police officers from across the Twin Cities who'd come to honor the memory of my youngest brother. It was all so surreal. Our car seemed to move in slow motion as my mind forever captured the grief-stricken expressions on each of their faces. Firefighters, citizens and their children lined the streets as well—it was a procession befitting a dignitary.

Eric's fellow officers had stood guard at each end of the table that held the urn at the visitation the evening before, and they continued to do so as mourners entered the church for the memorial service. At Amy's request, his brothers and sisters in uniform remained at the cemetery with her and the kids after everyone else had left—even family. I remember pulling from the embrace of an officer who told me, "Don't worry, ma'am; we have his watch covered." He also let me know that the

Roseville P.D. would make sure Amy and the kids were always taken care of.

It's an odd maxim—the one that says God never gives us more than we can handle. I disagree. It has been my experience that some families are on the receiving end of far more than they can deal with. I believe it's how they come out of the ordeal that matters. As a student in developmental psychology my first year of grad school, I learned that the goal of any stressful life event is to emerge from it strong enough to handle the next physical or emotional trauma—that part of grief and recovery is building resiliency. I remember watching the slide show, *The Interview with God,* over and over again while Eric was sick. A woman I worked with had sent it to me. She had the best attitude. *Maybe I need a little more of that kind of positivity,* I thought. Though I considered myself to be optimistic, I was also a bit too much of a realist. I was feeling tired and worn down.

Two weeks prior to Eric's death, Debbie shared with us that Andrea had been diagnosed with a brain tumor. She'd been vacationing that summer and had "symptoms" that she'd not wanted to share with the family because we were all so consumed and stressed by Eric's illness. It had gotten bad enough that she and Johnny went back to see her doctors at Johns Hopkins. Her brain surgery was scheduled for December 6, the day before my forty-ninth birthday. I don't remember much about my birthday that year, but I do remember three things from those weeks leading up to Christmas. The first was the phone call from Debbie that neurosurgeons had successfully removed a malignant mass from Andrea's brain—a *medulloblastoma,* a high-grade, fast-growing brain tumor. The second was a trip I made to the local mall sometime between my birthday and Christmas. I picked up a special ornament that I'd had engraved to hang on our Christmas tree that year in memory of Eric: "When someone you love becomes a memory, that memory becomes a treasure." There were flutists performing Christmas carols for the entertainment of the busy shoppers. The last bars of "Joy to the World" faded out, and they began to play "Amazing Grace" as I walked to the counter to pick up the ornament. *Since when is "Amazing Grace" a holiday song?* I thought. The lyrics rang out in my head. It was easy to follow along as I'd sung it a few weeks earlier with the other mourners at Eric's funeral. It was the last song of his service—the recessional as we left the church. "The Lord has promised good to me; His Word my hope secures; He will my shield and portion be as long as life endures." The saleswoman handed me the ornament to inspect before she placed it in the bag. My eyes were so filled with tears, it distorted into an unrecognizable blur. I barely managed to avoid a dreaded and almost-certain spillover onto the glass display case and hurried from the shop.

The third thing I remember was sending out my last ever family Christmas letter—asking those who received it, that if we should perhaps meet in the coming year, to ask me about my amazing brother. I didn't mention Andrea's brain surgery. I couldn't even bring myself to type those words.

CHAPTER 18: DOWN CAME THE RAIN

I should have planned something special for New Year's with the family, but my heart just wasn't in it. The holidays had left me numb and exhausted. After removing the ornaments and lights from our tree within those first days of 2007, I retreated downstairs for some solitude and time on the Internet. The computer in the basement was just as I'd left it. Piles of documents I'd printed sat next to it on the desk. A coffee mug and wine glass peeked out from the sea of my haphazard research.

I forced my weary eyes to stay focused on the computer screen and typed "familial adenomatous polyposis" into the search bar. I was dumbstruck by the volume of information related to FAP that had accumulated on the World Wide Web since my mother had died in 1997. Our "pesky colon" problem was all over the Internet. Whether a result of the information explosion that had occurred the previous decade, or the new research coming out of the field of medical genetics—shared instantly around the world among scientists and physicians studying inherited cancer syndromes—I didn't know. Whatever the case, it left me with the feeling we were entangled in something that was suddenly moving faster than we could keep up with. Had my siblings been aware of this new information? How much were they sharing with one another about their treatment plans and preventative care? I wasn't sure.

Frustrated, I continued to scroll down through the multitude of entries on the screen. It didn't take long to find journal entry after journal entry and abstract after abstract of new information related to our syndrome. I discovered that there were several variants of familial adenomatous polyposis, which made the disease even more complex than I had realized. I came across a number of studies describing elevated cancer risks *outside* of the colon, or *"extra colonic manifestations."* I pulled up a page from a Mayo Clinic site that referred to a link between stomach polyps, gastric cancers, and FAP. Not surprisingly, that connection stopped me in my tracks.

Feeling both overwhelmed and fueled by anger, I typed the keywords "brain lesions and familial adenomatous polyposis" into the search engine and scrolled down the screen.

And there it was: Turcot syndrome and medulloblastoma. Turcot's, or mismatch repair cancer syndrome, was associated with FAP. I'd never heard of it. I pressed my fingers to my temples as my eyes flew across the page. *My God,* I thought, *this can't be possible.* I took a deep breath and tried to ignore the heavy ache in my chest. I kept reading.

An editorial published in the late '90s referenced how dramatically the understanding of FAP had expanded over the last decade. *Yes,* I thought, *we've been brought up to speed rather quickly ourselves.* Another hour into my research, I came across a scholarly website that had been updated as recently as the October prior to Eric being diagnosed. It was called GeneReviews and included information on Familial

Adenomatous Polyposis and its variants. It provided a detailed look at the genetic mutation that five of my parents' children and seven of their grandchildren had inherited.

While scrolling through the website, I came across a table that laid out the lifetime risks of extra-colonic cancers in those with FAP. The site of the cancer, the type, and the additional risk faced by carriers of the APC gene were listed in no special order that I could determine.

Small bowel cancer is generally rare, affecting 0.2% of people in their lifetime; however patients with FAP are at a greater than 20-fold risk, particularly in the duodenum—the portion nearest the stomach. FAP carriers also had a slightly higher risk of developing stomach cancer. *Of course*, I thought, *Eric's "rare" stomach cancer.* Brain malignancies, usually medulloblastomas, were also more common in FAP patients. I immediately thought of Andrea. Then I scrolled down to a word that I'd not heard for over thirty-eight years: hepatoblastoma. Liver cancer. Hepatoblastoma is a one-in-a-hundred thousand cancer, but it occurs at a markedly higher rate (just under 1 in 100) in persons with FAP—most often in boys and typically within the first three years of life.

My thoughts drifted to Markie, lying in the casket in his blue suit, his eyes closed forever. I'd finally found the monster that killed him. It wasn't some boogeyman hiding in my closet—it was this damned DNA debris field known as the APC mutation. Markie'd had the mutated gene. We just didn't know it. Not even the doctors had made that connection in 1969. I thought of Karen in Texas. Did she know? If she did, why hadn't she said anything?

My mind hurtled back to the kitchen table conversation I'd had with my grandmother Evelyn in 1970, as she recalled that she'd thought there "might be something wrong" with my mother's family.

I looked down at my trembling hands. They shook so violently, I couldn't possibly type. I needed to take a break to try to calm my mind. I rose from my chair, and with one swift, violent sweep of my arm, sent the papers, coffee mug, and wine glass flying. The sound of shattering glass caused Bill to shout from the living room upstairs, "Hey, what the heck is going on down there?" I picked my way carefully through the broken glass and ascended the steps to the door leading to the basement. I made sure it was closed tightly. Then I went back downstairs, sat in the swivel chair, and started to wail. It was the wounded, guttural sound of pure heartbreak. I didn't want my kids to hear me. To hear such a thing is to relinquish all hope. Then the tears started to flow. I was surprised there were any left.

Suddenly the days of visits to Dr. Schultz were the "good old days"—days when our primary concern was the potential of a future colostomy. I missed his straight talk and connection to our family. We'd had no idea just how bad this mutation really was. It was as if the annoying, pain-in-the ass cousin you'd learned to live with had become a ruthless tormentor silently targeting those you love.

Then the panic started to set in. My fear was that our inherited polyposis wasn't just a colorectal syndrome, but a pre-cancerous state that would require even more vigilance on our part. I looked again at the percentages—even with the increased risk for cancers in other sites, the overall risk was still very low. But members of my family had been diagnosed with three of the rarest types—liver, stomach, and brain. Either those percentages were way off, or something else was going on.

The genetic test for the APC gene mutation hadn't become available to doctors until the mid-1990s. Would any of this knowledge have made a difference had we known in the '70s and '80s? How might my siblings and I have handled knowing all this back then? Would we have rushed our young children to the emergency room every time they had a stomachache? Or a headache?

The Interview with God spun in my head, "...that by thinking anxiously about the future, they forget the present, such that they live in neither the present or the future."

CHAPTER 19: **EXPRESSION**

Distressed by the most recent information we'd discovered about our family's inherited polyposis syndrome, Lisa, Marcie, and I decided to be tested again for the gene mutation. The test I'd had in 1999 was only 80 percent exclusionary because it failed to compare my DNA with that of any of my affected relatives. But by December of 2006, two of my family members with FAP had DNA samples on record at the University of Minnesota. It not only identified them as carriers of the APC mutation, but it specified exactly where the mutation was located on the chromosome itself. This time, the test would be much more definitive in determining—finally—if we carried it. And this time, unlike the test in 1999, I would meet with Dr. Richards as part of the genetic counseling. It would be two or three weeks before the results came back. In the meantime, I focused my energies on supporting my sister Debbie and her family.

The results of our genetic tests came back in early January. As I walked down Church Street toward the depressingly familiar red brick building that housed the cancer clinic on the University of Minnesota campus, I thought about the scientists in the late '80s that had laid the foundation for the discovery of the APC gene mutation. Dr. Richards and his team of scientists had been part of the race to find the exact location of the anomaly on chromosome 5, but they'd been beaten to the punch by two other research groups in the US who'd first honed in on the precise gene responsible for familial adenomatous polyposis. But Dr. Richards's kitchen-table prediction had proven true—it appeared that the same gene was likely to be involved in both sporadic and hereditary colon cancers.

I knew through my own research that more than fifty inherited cancer syndromes and the genes that cause them had been identified. The prevalence of FAP, in particular, has been estimated at 1 in 5,000 to 1 in 30,000 live births. It's considered a rare disease and accounts for less than 1 percent of all colorectal cancers diagnosed in the U.S. It's also nearly 100 percent penetrant. That means that virtually all carriers of the gene will, at some point, exhibit characteristics of it (like colorectal polyps, osteomas, lipomas, and freckles on the retina). Inherited disorders with that kind of penetration are extremely rare in the general population, which is why they are of special interest to researchers.

What that knowledge didn't tell me was why our family, given such a slight increase in risk for APC gene mutation carriers, had also been hit with exceedingly rare liver, stomach, and brain cancers. That was the one critical question I was determined to have answered.

A genetic counselor met with me to give me my test results before I met with Dr. Richards:

FAMILIAL ADENOMATOUS POLYPOSIS-APC KNOWN FAMILIAL MUTATION SEQUENCING RESULTS: NO FAMILIAL MUTATION DETECTED. *It is our understanding that this individual has a positive family history of Familial Adenomatous Polyposis (FAP). Previous molecular analysis performed in our laboratory of this individual's affected family member identified a deletion mutation 3202_3205delTCAA in exon 15 of the APC gene. Our molecular analysis of Laura Kieger's DNA did not identify the familial deletion mutation in the APC gene. These results indicate that Laura Kieger has not inherited the familial APC mutation.*

Those results felt final. I didn't carry the mutated gene. And because the gene was dominant, I also could not have passed it on to my three children. I was sure Bill and the kids would find the news comforting. I could hardly grasp the good news. I was angry. I wanted answers.

Sitting in his black, high-back swivel chair, Dr. Richards listened intently as I told him about Andrea's Turcot syndrome and Eric's rare stomach cancer. I shared a crudely drawn family pedigree chart with him, updated since my first genetic test. He wasn't surprised that I had questions.

According to Dr. Richards, mutations can "vary in their expressivity," which means that the severity of the symptoms can differ from person to person. It was the expressivity of our genetic mutation that I wanted to know more about. How could one very specific genetic mutation shared by members of my family "express" differently? Same family, same gene mutation, same "address" of the mutation, different cancer sites, different outcomes.

What I learned was there can be many different versions or variants of a given gene. The different versions of the gene are called alleles. There are nineteen alleles associated with our mutation address, Codon 1068. Different alleles of a gene "code" for the same trait, but they may manifest themselves in different ways. For example, the gene for eye color contains the instructions governing eye pigment, but the specific color is determined by the particular alleles one has. Everyone has the same number of chromosomes and genes, but each person's genetic code has a unique combination of alleles. This infinite potential for variation explains why we can all have extremely similar genomes, yet still have vast differences in characteristics and features.

I knew from my own research the previous month that a deletion mutation on Codon 1068 was what doctors might refer to as "classic" FAP. It governed the polyp "burden"—or the sheer number of polyps that might be found during an exam. Our particular mutation indicated a higher likelihood that ophthalmologists would find CHRPE, or the "freckles in the eye" marker. The 1068 mutation also presents an increased risk for the expression of Gardner's, a syndrome often manifesting in osteomas of the jaw and subcutaneous cysts like those my nieces had suffered as children.

I left Dr. Richard's office understanding that there can be great inconsistency in how familial polyposis disease is expressed, even among first-degree relatives who share the same mutation. Environmental and other genetic factors may play a role, as does "chance." While I could appreciate this, it was hard for me to accept. You can't control chance.

CHAPTER 20: SAYING GOODBYE

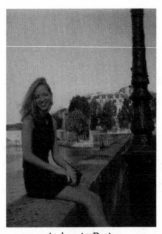

Andrea in Paris

With Andrea, as with Eric, there came the roller coaster of good news and bad news along with a lot of hope and prayer. The cancer in her brain hadn't been found in her cerebrospinal fluid, which was a very good thing. Andrea was also older than most medulloblastoma patients, which gave a boost to her five-year survival rate. We were optimistic about her chances. The aftermath of her surgery, however, proved devastating.

Neurologically speaking, she functioned as expected, but the radiation treatments coupled with intense physical therapy left her tired and frustrated with the pace of her recovery. Then one day in early March of 2007, Andrea collapsed into Debbie's arms without warning as they were preparing to leave for a therapy appointment. She died a few days later. The staggering post-op complications had overwhelmed her weakened body.

The call to Eric's wife, widowed just three months earlier, was terribly hard. Barely able to manage a whisper, I told her we would all understand if she couldn't be at the funeral.

A lengthy silence stretched over the line. Finally, she said, "I am so sorry... I'm glad you understand."

"Of course," I replied. We hardly expected Eric's wife or children to attend yet another funeral; they were already dealing with enough heartbreak. In spite of our own compounded grief, the rest of us would travel to Maryland to be with Debbie and her family and Andrea's husband Johnny— now a widower himself.

We flew into Dulles International. Debbie and Ron's friend Gail and her son Adam picked us up from the airport, so there was time to ask how everyone was holding up. "Numb" was the word I heard over and over again. A visitation would take place the following evening. My thoughts were thrust back to the pain of choosing photos for a video that played on a loop at Eric's visitation: Eric as a little boy standing proudly next to his banana seat bike; Eric in his catcher's gear, tagging an opposing player out at home plate; Eric looking handsome in his police uniform, his arm draped playfully over Cooper.

It's happening all over again, I thought. *What great injustice did our family perpetrate on the universe to deserve this?*

So many young people came together to remember Andrea—an undercurrent of "remember when" rippled through the memorial chapel. In our shared disbelief and profound sorrow, we all comforted Johnny and one another during the celebration of her life and upon that final, tearful goodbye as she was buried.

We'd been invited to a memorial service for the family organized by the residents of the senior assisted living center where Andrea worked. I wasn't sure what to expect. We arrived thirty minutes before the service was to start and were guided to an activity room complete with a large, black-lacquered piano. A charming elderly woman in a slightly askew hairpiece greeted us. She wore a floral dress that hung loosely from her thin shoulders and might have fit her perfectly many years before. She smiled and handed us each a program, taking our hands in hers—clad in gloves so white they looked like they'd never been worn. In a soft and slightly lilting southern accent, she said, "It's so nice that you've come so far to be with us today. Your family will all be seated in the front row, my dear." They were honored that we could join them in song and celebration to the wondrous love of Jesus, who'd prepared a place in Heaven for Andrea. I searched for the words to convey my gratitude for her thoughtfulness. What I couldn't seem to express verbally tumbled senselessly around in my head, so I just smiled and nodded.

The program was bright yellow—Andrea's favorite color—with small pictures of butterflies, flowers, and Jesus adorning the song lyrics. On the cover were the words, "When all my labors and trials are over and I am safe on the beautiful shore, Just to be near the dear Lord I adore will through the ages be glory for me."

Fred, a resident with a slow gait and wistful tenor sang a solo—"Precious Lord, Take My Hand"—accompanied by Geneva the pianist, who made sure the sheet music was at just the right height before she placed her long, dark fingers on the piano keys. Following Fred and Geneva's performance, the residents shared their individual precious memories of Andrea. They came forward one by one and proclaimed both their Christian faith and their love and admiration for my sweet niece. Several steadied themselves with canes; others held the microphone while seated in their wheelchairs. It was truly Andrea's moment—heartfelt and symbolic of who she was and how deeply she'd touched those around her.

One of the shared memories came from a woman named Margaret. She referred to Andrea as "Miss Andrea," and the two had a special bond. They'd both trained as dancers in their youth and shared a love of jazz and tap dancing. Margaret described how wonderful it was when Andrea would take her by the hand, and the two of them would tap out a little routine, reminding each other, "heel-toe" then "tap and turn."

"Miss Andrea always made me feel special," she said. "She was family to me, like a granddaughter. And now she sits at the table with the Lord. I know I will see her again soon."

As the visiting pastor began the sermon, I reached into my purse. There, folded up inside a zippered pocket was a piece of paper I'd been given by my father's best friend Marvin at Eric's funeral. On it he'd written, "Laura, I can't remember where I first read this, but it was written by a minister whose wife had died. I thought it was fitting for Eric." I unfolded the piece of paper and read the words in silence:

"A ship sails, and I stand watching till she fades on the horizon and someone at my side says, 'she is gone.' Gone where? Gone from my sight, that is all. She is just as large now as when I last saw her. Her diminished size and total loss from my sight is in me, not in her. And just at the moment when someone at my side says she is gone, there are others who are watching her coming over their Horizon and other voices take up a glad shout, 'There she comes!' That is what dying is...a horizon and just the limit of our sight. Lift us up, O Lord, that we may see further."

As I read the passage, I thought again of my mother's death the night of the wedding in 1997. She had gone from our sight, but I knew my father was on the far horizon waiting for her. And for a brief moment, I felt better knowing they both were there waiting for all of us, and had raised up a glad shout for Eric and for Andrea.

A day or two later, Debbie and I went to Johnny and Andrea's townhome to pick up a few items that Johnny thought Debbie would want: some jewelry and things from Andrea's childhood. I'd never been to the townhouse—they'd bought it as newlyweds just twenty-one months earlier. As we opened the front door and stepped into the living room, a corner unit immediately stood out. A number of its shelves were reserved for pictures of Andrea with her cousins, aunts, and uncles from Minnesota. Vacation pictures from Disneyworld and Paris in 2001. Photographs from Marcie and Jonathan's wedding in South Beach in 2003. It was an honored place in her Maryland home dedicated to her favorite memories with us. There it was, right in front of me. My fear that distance and time would chip away at her connectedness to the family ended at that very moment. Andrea hadn't left us behind. We had always been part of her busy life.

On the way to Baltimore-Washington International Airport, the swoosh-click, swoosh-click sound of the windshield wipers drowned out the radio program we were listening to. I was in the backseat with my suitcase, dreading leaving my devastated sister and brother-in-law behind. My mind drifted to the demands I had to deal with once home. Like finding auction items for Eric's fundraiser. And putting some pressure on Kelsey to make a final college decision. She had a couple of places in mind, but hadn't yet figured out where she wanted to go. I tried to be excited for her, but the mere thought of all that activity made me cringe. This time around was so different than it had been with Alex three years earlier. Back before we were broken. But mundane tasks were always the perfect anesthetic to anguish; when you piled them up, you could—at least temporarily—not feel or think and just do. Friederich Nietzsche summed it up when he said, "Haste is universal because everyone is in flight from himself."

A few miles from BWI my cell phone rang. It was Alex calling to let me know he was a finalist in a healthcare entrepreneurial competition and had been accepted to the University of Iowa's Summer Undergraduate Research program. I wanted to share his exciting news with Debbie and Ron, but it didn't seem the right time. Instead, I quietly told him how excited we were and that we'd try to visit him at the conclusion of the program. We said our goodbyes, and I flipped my cell phone shut. He'd be taking the Medical College Admissions Test (MCAT) later in the spring or early fall and thought being part of a research project as an undergrad would strengthen his application to medical school. I smiled to myself, proud mom thoughts running through my mind. He was working hard to achieve his goals, but there was still a long road ahead of him.

The airport was more crowded than I was accustomed to. Maybe the rain was backing up departures. Maybe it was because we were flying out on a Sunday. Whatever it was, security lines were long. Military servicemen and women crowded the airport, easily identified in their green camouflage and occasional dress uniforms. BWI was near several military bases, colleges, military contractors, and federal agencies, so their presence made sense. They all had somewhere to be.

My thoughts wandered while watching the conveyor belt carry my things toward the scanner. Memories of the backyard deck where we'd learned the "correct" way to eat Maryland crabs with Andrea and Johnny; watching Andrea walking down the aisle at her wedding; the ceramic Christmas village centerpieces that Debbie had been saving for her now and forever collecting dust in the basement—centerpieces she and Johnny would never use at their own holiday dinner table.

"Ma'am, excuse me, but you need to move forward."

I turned toward the voice. A nice looking young man stood behind me, waiting for me to pick up my personal items—now scanned and backing up the belt. Behind him stood several men and women in uniform, their backs perfectly straight and their eyes on me. I looked down at my stockinged feet and remembered where I was. Before I turned to recover my possessions, I said in the strongest voice I could muster, "I'm sorry. I came here for my niece's funeral, and I don't want to leave my sister."

The young man lowered his head slightly and took a deep breath before he responded, "I'm so sorry; take all the time you need."

I took another five to ten seconds to gather myself and slowly walked to gather my shoes and carry-on items. Everyone around me let me have that moment—even in the security line at a busy airport. Complete strangers, all with their own reasons to push through that line as fast as possible. But they all chose to be kind. No one said, "Hey lady, step it up," or, "What the hell are you doing standing there, I have a plane to catch."

There is a poem by Naomi Shihab Nye called "Kindness" from her book *The Words Under the Words: Selected Poems.* The experience at BWI reminded me of how she described the often lonely and desolate landscape of grief—that in order to know kindness you must also know deep sorrow. The people standing in line at the airport waiting for me to pull myself together had all almost certainly also wandered that landscape between sorrow and kindness. It's part of the frailty that holds us together as humans. Acts of kindness can help heal our grief. Even simple gifts like the poem Marvin had given me at Eric's funeral in the hopes that it would lift my spirits. And it had.

Much like the card and note my friend Monica had sent after Eric died that I'd left sitting on my desk at home. I'd been so busy, I hadn't had a chance to read it before I had to leave for yet another funeral. In it she wrote, "I once read that grief is an amalgam of emotions dependent on the circumstances: sadness, fear, anger, relief, and as such, frequently coupled with exhaustion. I think that's what makes it so uncontrollable and so frightening in and of itself. Any emotion can pop up at any moment—it's beyond one's control. The best one can do is *feel it through.*"

The coming months were going to be filled with emotional moments for the family. In April, Sergeant Eric Christensen would be posthumously awarded the Distinguished Service Award from the Minnesota Chiefs of Police Association. His wife, son, and daughter would be there to accept the award in honor and memory of my brother. There was going to be a benefit to raise money for a scholarship fund for students interested in becoming police officers. And Kelsey would be graduating from high school in June.

Feel it through, I told myself. Emotions might pop up at any moment. In *that* moment, I felt only detached. It was easier to tell people that the family was "fine," when the truth was that we were broken. I felt my faith slipping along with my energy. I didn't want to talk to people because they asked questions that I didn't have the answers to. But "feeling it through" would have to be enough, because, yes, any emotion can pop up at any time.

When I was a little girl, I'd stand in front of the refrigerator in our house on Shryer and read the Serenity Prayer. It seemed so simple. Control. I spent so much time trying to control every outcome, thinking if I could just anticipate potential disaster I could stay one step ahead of it or somehow keep it at bay. The problem was that I was just a powerless, anxious little kid. I was too young to understand the Serenity Prayer. I didn't have "the wisdom to know the difference" then.

I replaced the verse that Marvin had given me with the note from Monica, tucking it carefully into my wallet. I had a feeling that I'd be regularly reaching for it to help me through the emotional, physical, and spiritual game of chutes and ladders to come in the months—and perhaps years—ahead.

PART THREE:

The Road Ahead

CHAPTER 21: **FREEFALL**

Heading into the summer of 2007, my emotions continued to ricochet between disbelief, detachment, and anger, all accompanied by an unyielding exhaustion. Kelsey took the brunt of my apathy during her pre-college summer planning. Though I could have been a big help to her while she was immersed in new student orientation, checking out her dorm, and figuring out her fall semester schedule, I was instead distant and disengaged.

I was a lost cause. I had trouble reaching out to friends and became a bit of a recluse—not my normal self. Debbie wasn't up to coming to Minneapolis for the graduation party, which Kelsey completely understood. I once read somewhere that when we grieve for the dead we leave the living behind. It was something I knew all too well. And it scared the hell out of me.

Alex left Minnesota after the ceremony and celebration to resume his involvement in the summer undergraduate research program at the University of Iowa. There would be a presentation later that summer, which Bill and I planned to attend. We'd never been to Iowa City and since the timing coincided with our wedding anniversary, we decided it would make for a nice long weekend. And I'd convinced Bill that Galena, Illinois, where my mother's Aunt Adele was buried, was worth a visit as it was only a couple of hours from the University campus. Not to mention, I desperately needed a road trip.

I'd asked—no, *begged*—my parents to take me with them to bury my Auntie Del in 1969. They'd given me a firm "no" that put a quick end to my pleading. They would take her body to Galena. That's what my Auntie Del wanted—to be buried near her parents and sister Pauline in the town where she grew up.

Initially, I had very little to base my search for Adele's burial site on. I knew she would be buried in a Catholic cemetery. That much was a given. Coincidentally (or perhaps not), during my Internet research over the previous year, I'd entered my great-aunt's name into the search bar and happened upon a genealogist's work that had been conducted inside of the cemeteries of Jo Daviess County, Illinois. From there it didn't take me long to find the records of a St. Mary's Cemetery in Galena. Someone with the genealogy society had physically walked through the cemetery, conscientiously taking down the names and dates on every headstone, along with the location of the graves. I scanned the records looking for the surname of Ortscheid. Miraculously, there it was. I'd found my Aunt Adele's cemetery plot. I couldn't believe my luck.

Bill and I drove through southeastern Minnesota and into Wisconsin, taking the longer scenic route. I'd forgotten just how charming the small towns that dotted the landscape along the Mississippi river could be. I'd traveled through many of those same small towns as a child—pit stops on the way to somewhere else—places to fill the station wagon's gas tank or to buy a map because we were lost. If my parents were in a good mood (meaning we didn't need a map) they'd buy us a bottle of pop for the road ahead.

We followed State Highway 35 along the river for as long as we could, traveled east through Platteville and then turned south again toward Galena, catching State Highway 20 towards town. Night was falling, and Bill asked me where we were staying in Galena. I hadn't given it much advance thought but had jotted down a couple of places along with their phone numbers. The first one on my short list had a room for us. The hotel was right off of Highway 20 and Spring Street and had a woodsy, wilderness theme. To my disappointment though, the hotel was outside downtown Galena, recently cited in *LIFE* magazine's *America the Beautiful* edition as one of the "100 Places to See in Your Lifetime." There would be no late night stroll down the quaint main streets of Galena that night—we were too far from the historic city center.

The next morning, as Bill was putting our suitcase in our car, I stopped at the front desk to speak to the concierge. I explained that we didn't have a lot of time, but asked if he could help me find St. Mary's cemetery.

The young man smiled and pointed toward one of the windows. "You won't have to drive far," he said. "It's right across the street."

My heart raced as I rushed back to our room to tell Bill. I practically dashed through the traffic on Highway 20 and once inside the wrought iron gates, promptly kicked off my sandals and walked barefoot among the headstones and markers. I couldn't help but notice the lovely rolling hills below the cemetery. Green grass, sunshine, and bright blue sky. When I came across an Ortscheid grave I knew I was close, and there in section 2, lot 18 I found her. Adele Ortscheid Baker. Born 1892. Died 1969. Her plot was next to her sister's; I was happy to see that. She was also situated near her parents. I sat down beside her grave and looked out toward the hills, thinking, *This is a nice view, Auntie Del.* Bill wandered among the headstones in the distance, giving me some much needed space and time. Memories of growing up with this woman as my surrogate maternal grandmother came rushing back, including all the love and support she'd provided for our family.

Auntie Del had always made me feel special. She would arrive at our house on Shryer and call for me, the remnants of her German accent giving my name a romantic sounding "Lara" lilt. I remembered driving with my mom to the Sears Roebuck Catalog Outlet in Har Mar Mall to pick up a gift she'd ordered for my seventh birthday. Not only did she give me seven crisp one-dollar bills wrapped in gold paper inside of a card, she bought me a doll that I was desperately hoping for. Not just an ordinary baby doll, but a stop-my-beating-heart, beautiful doll with chocolate brown hair and eyes, wearing a fancy pink chiffon dress, bonnet, and booties. I opened the box and gasped then squealed with delight. That doll was a treasured connection to her that comforted me long after Auntie Del had passed. I was only ten when she died, but she'd had a profound impact on me. She taught me about hard work and responsibility, keeping the faith, and how not to be afraid.

I kissed the tips of my fingers and pressed them to the etching of her name in the stone, promising to return someday.

We continued on our way to the University of Iowa, traveling east toward Dubuque, then south along the Iowa border with Illinois, and then once again following the

Mississippi River. The 2007 Summer Undergraduate Research Conference would be well under way by the time we arrived. Alex was anticipating our arrival, though he'd said, "It's not a big deal Mom; it's basically a poster, and we talk to people about our research." Once Bill and I found our hotel and unpacked, we made our way to the auditorium where the conference was taking place.

In Iowa City, it's all about the Hawkeyes. The campus was the main draw in town. I immediately fell in love with it. We took our time traversing the campus, stopping along the way to take pictures and get a feel for what Alex's summer experience must have been like. He'd made some new friends—most of them attended colleges in the Midwest and were in their junior or senior years. After the conference he'd return to Drake University in Des Moines to finish up his senior year, but not before he took the MCAT back in the Twin Cities.

When we arrived at the conference site we were greeted by Alex's mentor, an MD PhD from Stanford, who immediately asked, "So, which one of you is the scientist in the family?" That was amusing because it wasn't the first time someone had asked Bill and me that question. We explained that neither one of us could take the credit.

I was stunned to learn that Alex's team had focused its research project on genetics—specifically the genetics of cancer. Their poster presentation was titled, "Examining The Role of Chromatin Regulators in Cancer Pre-Disposition"—those cancers that appeared to be hereditary, or cancer syndromes caused by genetic mutations similar to that which my family had inherited.

I listened with great interest to their explanations of the science behind their project but wished I had a translator with me—most of what they shared went over my head, despite all of my own research on the subject. As I wandered around the auditorium speaking to so many bright, young minds about their studies and projects, it dawned on me that I was looking at the next generation of doctors and medical researchers. Some of them might discover treatment breakthroughs and potentially even cures for some of the most devastating and debilitating diseases.

In the course of my many months of research, I'd discovered that it can take as many as seventeen years for basic research to move from the scientific "bench" to the patient's bedside (or into the hands of the practicing physician who treats the patient.) Further complicating this delay are "silos" between institutions—wherein non-integrated systems, proprietarily held information, and a lack of funding can prevent effective collaboration and information sharing. In essence, valuable research and knowledge that could save lives and improve patient care gets tangled up in technical, financial, and bureaucratic webs. I could only hope that some of the great minds in that auditorium might one day focus on translational research and clinical care, and help to dissolve those barriers between "lab bench and patient bedside."

Alex's fourth grade creative writing assignment came into my mind, *I think a Medical Researcher has the most important job...*

And there he was participating in a research program that had brought him full circle.

CHAPTER 22: ERA OF THE GENOME (1990-2003)

In 1990, the National Institute of Health and the Department of Energy published a plan for the first five years of an expected fifteen-year endeavor known as the Human Genome Project. That undertaking developed additional technologies for rapidly analyzing DNA and sought to map and sequence the genomes of fruit flies, mice, and ultimately humans. The goal was to provide researchers with powerful tools to understand the genetic factors in human disease, paving the way for new strategies for diagnosis, treatment, and prevention.

Around the time that the plan for the Human Genome Project was published, the first evidence of the BRCA1 gene was discovered. BRCA1 (Breast Cancer gene 1) is a "tumor suppressor gene," which normally produces a protein that prevents cells from growing and dividing out of control as occurs in cancer. Researchers eventually identified more than 1,000 mutations of the BRCA1 gene, many of them associated with increased risks for breast and ovarian cancers in women. This important discovery now enabled BRACA testing for high-risk individuals. Genes associated with Wilms' tumour, Li

Fraumeni syndrome, neurofibromatosis, von Hippel-Landau disease and retinoblastoma were also located.

In the early '90s, around the same time the BRCA 1 gene was found, the genetic mutation that causes FAP was discovered. Only three years after Dr. Richards and his nurse drew our blood at our mother's kitchen table, two teams from the U.S., one from Utah and another from Baltimore, published their findings on the same day—August 9, 1991, twenty-two years to the day that Markie died. The gene on chromosome 5 now had a name as well: APC or Adenomatous Polyposis Coli.

The identification of APC would change everything for familial polyposis syndrome families and the guidelines for managing their care. APC is a tumor suppressor gene much like BRCA1. Tumor suppressor genes normally protect our cells from becoming cancerous. The mutation in the APC gene that my family inherited results in "switching APC off"—leaving once healthy cells exposed to a relentless bombardment of signals telling them to keep growing—ultimately leading to the formation of tumors.

That same day, August 9, 1991, the New York Times featured news of the APC discovery in the article "Doctors Link Gene to Colon Cancer" by Natalie Angier. In it she describes that the newly detected gene should allow doctors to identify those with an inborn predisposition to colon cancer and that people found to carry the defective gene could then be screened with heightened diligence. Dr. Henry Lynch was quoted in the New York Times article announcing, "This is a major milestone in colorectal cancer research that will echo around the world." He went on to say, "I haven't done too well in treating patients with advanced colon cancer, and neither have any of my colleagues. The most important thing is to detect the cancer early, when it's at a curable stage, and that's what this work is all about."

In April of 2003, under budget and more than two years ahead of schedule, researchers successfully completed the Human Genome Project. To date, it has allowed for the discovery of more than 1,800 genetic diseases. As a result of this massive effort, today's researchers can find a gene suspected of causing an inherited syndrome in a matter of days, rather than the years that were necessary before the genome sequence was in hand. Nobel Laureate James D. Watson stated, "Never would I have dreamed in 1953 that my scientific life would encompass the path from DNA's double helix to the three billion steps of the human genome. But when the opportunity arose to sequence the human genome, I knew it was something that could be done—and that must be done. The completion of the Human Genome Project is a truly momentous occasion for every human being around the globe."

The rapid expansion of the Internet in the late '90s allowed it to become a repository for the data compiled by those involved with the Human Genome Project. This enabled it to be readily available and accessed by virtually anyone, serving to rapidly increase the pace of medical discovery worldwide. Basic cancer research was now leading more quickly and directly to the translation of important findings into actionable information for patients. The advent of the Internet was a flash point igniting and rapidly shaving months and perhaps even years off of the painful time it took information to get from "bench to bedside."

It had been a confluence of several of these key events in the scientific and medical communities that contributed to my family's challenging journey of learning about and living with the disease called Familial Adenomatous Polyposis. Thanks to the advanced laboratory techniques developed in the '80s that allowed for DNA to be more easily synthesized and analyzed, the discovery of the FAP causing APC gene mutation in 1991 leading to a genetic test for the mutation, the completion of the Human Genome Project in 2003, and the surging influence and information-sharing capabilities of the Internet and World Wide Web, there are now answers available to questions we didn't even know to ask.

The advances leading to a greater understanding of familial polyposis and the APC gene mutation's vicious grip had taken many generations. We, like countless others suffering from inherited cancer pre-disposition syndromes, had simply been snared in a constant and sometimes ugly game of catch-up. The seemingly endless journey so plagued with fits and starts was finally beginning to accelerate.

CHAPTER 23: THE DEEPEST THINGS INSIDE

In late August of 2007, we moved Kelsey into her dormitory at Winona State University. I remember it well because she was assigned to the women's-only dorm after submitting her housing application late in the assignment process. Her father was pleased with that outcome. It was pretty apparent she was a bit of an outlier compared to the other girls rooming on her floor. The Resident Advisors had each of them put their name on the outside of their door and then asked them to add pictures, a quote, or anything else that might reflect to visitors something about the young women living in that particular room. There were pictures of animals, famous actors and actresses, poems, and references to reaching for the stars and becoming the next great leader or humanitarian. Kelsey had no pictures and just this taped to her dorm room door: *The real measure of success is what you do with plan B.* That, I thought, was perfect for her. She'd not only inherited her dad's green eyes, she had also inherited my power of accurate observation. Having a plan B is about reality. From choosing her major, to researching which companies might offer the perfect internship opportunities, to figuring out how to stretch her budget, she always had a plan. And a back-up. She innately understood that people grow, plans change, and that the aspirations of a young adult are fluid. I wish I'd been that astute at eighteen.

We expected her back home again for Thanksgiving. I wanted a good holiday weekend, if that was even possible. After all, my sister Lisa and her husband Mark were due to be grandparents for the first time in the middle of November.

When my mother was dying in 1997, I'd take short breaks from the painful chaos that overshadowed her final days and walk down to the newborn nursery. That was at a time before you needed a security badge to wander the maternity ward. Seeing those little scrunched up faces wrapped tightly in their buntings never failed to lift my spirits. That's how I felt when I held Taylor Ann for the first time. She was a light during a difficult holiday.

I tried to reach out to Debbie and Ron and Eric's wife, Amy and their kids as often as I could. It wasn't easy. After Eric and Andrea died we all retreated to our figurative emotional corners. While working on a consulting project in December of 2007 and trying to figure out how I was going to grab a bite to eat while still meeting an early afternoon deadline, I happened to click on a story about a man whose daughter had died suddenly during a semester abroad. While living in a foreign country with limited healthcare options, a fast moving bacterial infection had taken her life. The girl's father talked about building resiliency and how he was still trying to come to grips with life without her and described it as his "new normal."

It was the first time I'd ever heard that expression used that way. It resonated with me because it acknowledged that things weren't—and never would be—the same as they had been, yet still implied getting on with life. I thought long and hard about my next move. Then I clicked on the "e-mail this story" button and sent it to Debbie. I hoped it wouldn't upset her because I was hardly in a position to offer advice or insight. A few hours later, she replied with a simple "thank you."

Sitting in my car on a cold evening in March of 2008, I stopped at our mailbox to grab the day's delivery. After turning into our driveway and closing the garage door behind me, I walked through the entryway and tossed the mail on the small table I'd positioned below an etched, mother-of-pearl mirror that had been my Auntie Del's. An unfamiliar reflection caught my eye. I needed to color my hair badly—faint streaks of gray were peeking through, which I supposed was inevitable given that I'd turned forty-nine the past December. I couldn't remember the last time I'd been physically active beyond a few tosses of snow from my front steps while shoveling and slogging through my day. My cross-country skis were gathering dust up in the attic, and I'd never really warmed to the idea of snowshoeing like Bill had. It had been several years since I'd downhill skied. Maybe we could go West come spring. I'd love for Addy to snowboard with her dad and me in Vail. We could start together on the green runs until she felt comfortable with the altitude and sheer physicality of mountain skiing and snowboarding.

I stared at myself in the mirror again. Who was that person? I pulled my gloves off one finger at a time and shuffled through the mail. Tucked in the stack, I discovered an envelope from Northwestern University Feinberg School of Medicine in Chicago. Alex had applied to a couple of medical schools the previous fall, and we'd spent the intervening months waiting to hear which schools would offer him a spot in their graduating class of 2012. I wasn't comfortable opening the letter myself, but I could barely contain my curiosity and excitement long enough to call and leave him a message. He called back right away, and the first words out of his mouth were, "Open it, Mom! What are you waiting for?"

I turned the envelope over and used my car keys to open it. The letter inside was signed by the Associate Dean for Admissions. I read the first line: "Dear Alexander, I am pleased to offer you a position in the incoming first year class at Northwestern University's Feinberg School of Medicine." I read the letter to him over the phone. He'd already been accepted at the University of Iowa so now it was decision time. I congratulated him and flipped my cell phone shut. Instinctively, I called to Bill who was sitting in our living room watching the evening news. "What day is it today?" I asked.

"March 3rd. Why?"

March 3, 2008. Exactly one year to the day that Andrea had passed away. My eyes came to rest on the last paragraph of the acceptance, "I look forward to seeing you...on August 25, 2008, when we will welcome you as a member of the class of 2012." August 25. Eric's birthday. The significance of those dates temporarily stunned me. After collecting my thoughts, I walked into the living room, swallowing the lump that had risen in my throat, and held the letter out to Bill.

Later that evening, overwhelmed with emotion, I sent an email to Debbie to share the news with her. I closed by saying, "I have to believe that there's some deeper meaning to all of this, or I would have trouble seeing light again."

In 2009, Pixar came out with a lovely little movie called *Up*. Addy and Bill were in agreement that we should go see it. High-end Disney animation coupled with a talking Golden Retriever sounded entertaining. My enthusiasm was more restrained, but I knew I should tag along. I'd enjoyed *Toy Story*—how much different could this movie be? Maybe ten minutes into the movie I was swept along by stirring scenes showing the unfolding relationship between husband and wife, Carl and Ellie. After Ellie dies, a grieving Carl finds her "My Adventure Book" and pages through it, finding that Ellie had documented the cherished moments—the small every day events that happen over a lifetime together. *How fitting,* I thought. *We all have an adventure book inside.*

Bill and I would be celebrating our 25th wedding anniversary that summer. I thought of Andrea and Johnny who would have been married four years that very month. My watery eyes spilled over. Tears coursed down my checks, and swiftly led to full-scale sobbing. I was a hot mess. Addy handed me the greasy napkin she'd been using to wipe the popcorn butter from her fingers. While thoughtful, one napkin wasn't going to help. She rested her hand on my arm, either to comfort me or as if to pull a lever to make it stop. But I couldn't stop. I jumped out of my seat and raced for the restroom. I stepped on Bill's toes in the process and sent his supersized lemonade flying from the cup holder. A real train wreck.

In the quiet calm of the bathroom stall, I reached into my purse and withdrew the note from Monica, still tucked away in my wallet after more than two years. "Any emotion can pop up at any moment—it's beyond one's control...the best one can do is feel it through." I loitered in the restroom for another fifteen minutes and pulled myself together, then walked out stopping at the concession stand for a bottle of water and an enormous stack of napkins. I ignored the look of disgust shot my way from the fifteen-year-old behind the counter and worked my way back to my seat. Bill didn't say a thing. Neither did Addy. I managed to stay until the very end and was rather proud of the fact.

Bill and Addy were quiet during the car ride home, perhaps sensing that I needed some time to be alone with my thoughts. The idea of an "adventure book"—a precious reminder of all of the events both trivial and profound that coalesce into this magical thing we call life—remained on my mind. As much as I tried not to devolve into grief or self-pity, the only thought I could manage was, *why are the pages so often filled with pain? Why is life sometimes so damn hard?* All around me, things seemed to be falling apart. Loved ones dying. Friends my age losing their jobs, health insurance, and savings due to the recession. Once-strong relationships at risk of flaming out. So many people that I loved were living those experiences. They, too, knew the kind of hurt that pulsates far beneath the surface, then returns in waves. *Like emotions that can pop up at any moment.*

Why is life so hard? I wondered again. It was while sitting in that quiet car on the way home from a kid's movie that a whisper of the answer came. Perhaps in some strange way it's *meant* to be hard—part of a complex but necessary design in which the random and unexpected can crush us in one moment and lift us up in the next. It's only because we experience great suffering that we can also know great joy. As Naomi Shihab Nye wrote: "before you know kindness as the deepest thing inside, you must know sorrow as the other deepest thing." One cannot exist without the other.

It was time to try to find that joy again.

It was then, with some trepidation, that I started planning a trip to Italy with Debbie and Marcie for May of the following year, 2010. Kelsey and her cousin would join Marcie and me during the first part of the trip, then the girls and I would meet Debbie and Ron in Rome while Marcie returned to the States. The time with Kelsey was important to me; I hoped I could make amends for some of the unfair and unwarranted emotional disappointments and wrongdoings she'd had to endure from me late in her senior year of high school.

My hesitation was in meeting with Debbie and Ron in Rome. I wasn't sure how ready Debbie would be to travel with her two nieces, both in their early twenties. Would memories of our Paris trip with Andrea in 2001 be overwhelming for her? As we communicated back and forth about apartment rentals and travel itineraries, I heard no hesitation in her voice, which was comforting. She even suggested we spend an afternoon in Rome taking a cooking class. I thought that Kelsey, a self-described "foodie" would enjoy the opportunity and readily agreed.

Between the Coliseum, the Spanish Steps, and the Vatican, the cooking class at *le Fate in Roma* was at the top of Kelsey's list. We took the train from Naples to Rome and once we found our rental apartment, quickly unpacked so we could familiarize ourselves with the neighborhood. A popular gelato shop was a few feet from our building, and we were almost directly across from a busy Italian restaurant. The male waiters there would follow the girls calling, "Bellissima!" as they moved out of striking distance. I was always just a few steps behind, and they would suddenly change their catcalls to "Oh, Mamma! How nice to see you as well." Italian men were exactly how other women had described them to me—rascals and flirts, albeit with the typical warmth of character of the Italian people.

We spent a full day with a local guide who happened to be from the United States. She'd followed a love interest to Rome and decided the city was a better match for her than the man she'd come for. She took us through the Pantheon and "old Roma" to see the ruins, as well as the Coliseum. We avoided the expensive shops in favor of the open-air markets, and the girls each fastened upon a short leather jacket as their must-have souvenir. Our apartment was ideally located—within walking distance to Piazza Navona, one of Rome's most treasured piazzas. For centuries, acrobats and jugglers have performed there, and it's still lively and bustling with artists and street performers. The quaint espresso cafes and fantastic people watching make it a favorite locale for travelers. In the center of the piazza is Bernini's famous fountain—La Fontana dei Fiumi erected in 1651. The centerpiece of the fountain is a tall Roman obelisk surrounded by four giants representing each of the great rivers: Ganges, Nile, Danube, and Plate.

The day of our Italian cooking class arrived, and the girls couldn't have been more excited. For me the idea of spending four hours in a kitchen was far from enjoyable, but I would be a good sport as it was a new experience for me. The full extent of my cooking education had consisted of my mother shooing me out of the kitchen and an eighth grade foods class, which was only slightly less aggravating than eighth grade sewing.

We rode the bus to the Trastevere neighborhood and arrived at Le Fate, a trattoria. The trattorias are traditionally family-owned, casual neighborhood restaurants found throughout all of Italy that serve fresh local food. "Delightful" is the word that came to my mind as my eyes scanned the small yet charming dining area. I asked Debbie the meaning of Le Fate, and she told me that it means "fairy."

We weren't seated for more than a few minutes before the Master Chef—our cooking instructor—came to introduce himself. Handsome and dressed in a black chef's coat, he reached out his hand to us and said, "I am Chef Andrea, and I welcome you to Le Fate."

At the mention of his name, I was stunned silent. I watched Debbie's expression, sensing one of those "moments" that Monica's note had warned me about. I waited for sadness to descend on the table, but it never really did. Debbie thanked him by name with a warm, genuine smile.

It would prove to be a good afternoon. I developed some patience and learned not be a total hindrance in the kitchen. We all had a lovely time. Making homemade pasta and squash blossoms and tiramisu with Chef Andrea was an adventure we would talk about for years to come.

It was a small, yet significant step toward our new normal.

CHAPTER 24: JOHNS HOPKINS BOUND

Around the time Bill and I were experiencing our third high school spring break, prom, and high school graduation, we'd also just celebrated Kelsey's college graduation—with honors—from Winona State University. Class of 2011. Though we were thrilled she would be coming back to the Twin Cities to start her professional career, Bill and I were trying to come to grips with the idea that her two-year plan included a move to another city with a milder climate. Winter wind chills would not follow her to Austin, Texas or perhaps San Francisco, California. Two years seemed right around the corner.

Addy's post-high school plans would take her five hours north and slightly west to the University of North Dakota. The thought of wearing a hooded parka and Sorel's six months out of the year didn't bother her, provided they were fashionable. Addy hadn't yet decided on a major, but she was absolutely certain that she wanted to be free of daily parental oversight. We were more than willing to oblige. I'd never met anyone as truly dedicated to the concept of "living for the moment" as my youngest child. And unlike her older sister, she never had need of a "plan B." She just adapted to whatever came her way.

My brother Butch was looking forward to driving to Minnesota for Addy's grad party and an extended month-long stay in the Cities to visit with family. A few days prior to making the trip, he called from Arizona and asked if I thought it was safe for him to travel. I wasn't sure what he meant, so I asked why he was concerned.

I could hear his wife Mary in the background shouting, "He's jaundiced! He's yellow!"

A knot tightened in my stomach. "What's going on, Butch?" I asked.

He told me he'd lost quite a bit of weight recently and had been low on energy. He'd gone to the doctor and his lab tests had raised several red flags. I knew how desperately he wanted to come home to Minnesota to see his grandsons, do a little fishing, and participate in Addy's graduation celebration. But driving all those miles while not feeling well didn't seem like the best idea to me.

"I'd rather you stay in Arizona and see your doctors," I said. "Figure out what's going on."

He did just that. Within a few weeks of that phone call, he learned that he had three small cancerous tumors in his upper GI tract—one near the head of his pancreas, one in his duodenum, and one in his biliary system. The jaundice was a symptom of an associated blockage.

The extra-colonic manifestations of familial polyposis. Again. Butch spent that summer recovering from a "modified Whipple" surgery and underwent a round of just-in-case chemotherapy. Fortunately, his cancers were found in the early stages, and his prognosis was good. It served as a reminder to all of us that maintaining the surveillance program of regular endoscopies and colonoscopies could result in early diagnosis and treatment. One of my gene mutation-carrying siblings had once been told by their doctor, "If you don't come in to see me on a regular basis, don't bother coming in at all."

Over the years, we'd come to understand the difficulties and challenges for doctors that come with treating familial polyposis patients. They want to help those under their care to stay ahead of the disease as much as their families do, but that is partly dependent on the patient's adherence to their exam schedules and prescribed treatment regimens. Doctors often develop strong bonds with patients who are carriers of a gene predisposing them to cancer. We'd been fortunate to have that with Dr. Schultz. I never once caught him checking his watch or felt rushed while I was in his office discussing the results of my annual exams. He would always take the time to ask how the family was doing. He even came to my mom's funeral, at which I thanked him for saving her life when I was thirteen with a warm hug.

In March of 2012, we were waiting to hear where Alex would be matched for his residency. Match Day was around the corner for Northwestern University's Feinberg School of Medicine graduates. The official announcements would occur in the middle of March at a local restaurant in downtown Chicago. If the students were really lucky, Match Day would coincide with St. Patrick's Day, and then a real party—complete with green beer and a green river running through the city— would ensue. Alex's interest was radiology, and had been his focus for the last two years of medical school. It was difficult for me to know he might wind up virtually anywhere in the country. Chicago had been so convenient for Bill and me to visit, and we'd really gotten to know the city. But we knew how important this was to him and how hard he'd worked to obtain a residency in radiology.

In the midst of all the excitement, Bill and Alex had decided to go to Breckenridge, Colorado to snowboard during spring break week. While they were away, I went to Andrea's online memorial to leave a message. Her friend Melissa had set up the online memorial and she and several of Andrea's friends all participated in an annual brain cancer 5K fundraiser every year since her death. I wondered how Johnny was doing and realized I hadn't been back to Maryland since the funeral. It had been five difficult years for the family, yet I could close my eyes and go back in an instant, the bagpipes playing as we stood at her gravesite.

I was in the middle of drafting an outline for a workplace satisfaction survey when my cell phone rang. It was Alex calling.

"Hey, aren't you on a chairlift somewhere enjoying your break?" I teased. The signal was surprisingly clear because he was, indeed, calling me from Breckenridge while sitting on a chairlift next to his dad.

"Mom, I know where I matched. I found out a few days early."

I could tell by the enthusiasm in his voice that he was pleased with the outcome of his match, even though he wasn't in the middle of a Chicago restaurant filled with medical students jumping around waving their envelopes in the air. I was anxious to hear.

"Johns Hopkins," he said, "I matched at Johns Hopkins. Can you believe it? I'll be going to Baltimore. But not until the summer of 2013. I'll be spending another year at Northwestern as a surgery intern before my residency starts."

There were a few things that I had to quickly wrap my head around. Our son—who'd once been caught streaking with his high school buddies across the football field at halftime of the Homecoming game wearing nothing but super hero masks, capes, and underwear—would soon be removing gallbladders and assisting with liver transplants.

Damn, I thought, *he's going to be great at that.* His 10th grade biology teacher had predicted it: "I've never seen a surgical incision so cleanly and effortlessly performed on a fetal pig by a sixteen year old student. Most of the kids just hack away."

And Johns Hopkins. *World-renowned* Johns Hopkins. Where Debbie and Andrea had been patients for years. Where another of my nieces was currently considering joining a clinical trial for her familial polyposis. Now Alex would be there, walking those same hallways as a physician. He might even be introduced to Debbie's doctors and the clinical staff that had loved and cared for Andrea in her final days. Honestly, it was a bit unreal.

These thoughts were still racing around my head when I faintly heard the words, "...and I just missed a tree yesterday coming down a fantastic run while trying to avoid a collision with a little kid. I'm telling you Mom, some of these snowboarder wannabes are out of control."

Drawing quickly back into our phone conversation, I congratulated him on his great news and played the mom card.

"You'd better be wearing your helmet," I said. I ended our conversation with, "I'm proud of you, kiddo."

I looked at the time on my desktop computer. I had forty-five minutes until my next meeting. I dialed Debbie's number. She didn't pick up. I left her a message to call me as soon as she could. Then I waited. Twenty excruciating minutes later my phone rang.

It was Debbie. "Hey sis, what's going on?"

"Are you sitting down?" I asked. "It's great news."

"That's good," she replied. "What's up?"

"I just got a call from Alex," I said. "He matched at Johns Hopkins for his residency. He'll be out in Baltimore the summer of 2013." I wondered if she could sense the relief in my voice to know he'd be close to family.

"Wait," she said, "let me put you on speaker phone so Ron can hear."

I gave them the news. "I just wanted to make sure you could help me out with making sure he eats; he can get caught up in his work and forget. And he might need help navigating the city. And—sorry—the occasional use of your vehicle. But he's a self-described low-maintenance guy. In fact, he likes to brag most of his possessions would fit into a small duffle bag. I just wanted to give you a heads up."

She sounded happy, with a fullness of heart I'd not heard since before everything came crashing down on us. "Not a problem, Laura. That's great news! And he can use the Mountaineer. Does he have a place to stay? We have the room here if he needs it. Even better, I'll talk with some of my connections at the hospital about the nearby neighborhoods.

And Johnny may have some ideas. A lot of the young doctors seem to gravitate toward Fells Point or Federal Hill..."

Looking back on the previous six years, I realized that feelings of hope had been creeping into my psyche again. I suddenly felt very grateful. Gratitude is hard when you're hurting. Many people had come in and out of our lives at just the right moments over the last several years, some of whom I'd failed to thank while I'd been otherwise "disconnected."

I stopped by the State Fairgrounds and had a cup of coffee with the owners of the Lunch Box, reintroducing myself because it had been so long since I'd even thought of spending a day at the fair. Starting in 2001 and every summer thereafter through 2011, they'd given jobs to my three kids (plus my niece and nephew). They worked the counter for those ten crazy days learning how a family business operates. The experience had taught our teenagers what it meant to show up for work on time, and how to work hard, and even how to have a little fun in the process. I laughed when they asked if I had more children in the pipeline.

I sent a handwritten "Thank you" card to Addy's senior-year art teacher, Ms. Moore. At the last parent-teacher conference before the school year ended, Ms. Moore had gushed about my daughter's creative potential and showed me a series of Mod Podge paper cards she'd made, each representing something important to her. I knew that no matter what was going on in Addy's life during her senior year, Ms. Moore's art class had been a sanctuary for her.

Feeling energized, I sent an email to Colleen, a manager at Allina Health, regarding Alex's path from emergency room volunteer, to dietary aide, to medical student, to doctor. I thanked her for being a great mentor to him. She ended her reply with, "Thank you for letting me know I made a difference, you made my day!"

Smiling, I shut down my computer and looked out the window. I thought once more about the note Monica had sent me back in March of 2007, the one I carried in my wallet to remind me that with grief, emotions can pop up at any time. I walked over to our dining room table where my purse was sitting and pulled out my wallet. It was still there, tucked between the laminated copy of my father's obituary and a business card from the Italian restaurant Le Fate. I unfolded the note and read it once more, but this time I didn't return it to my wallet. As transitional objects, I no longer felt as if I needed either the note or the obituary. I went to the master bedroom and reached down beneath the bed for the silver metal box that had once belonged to my parents. After carefully placing each of them inside, I pushed the box under the bed again and then hollered to our golden retriever, Huck, asking him if he wanted to go for a walk. I took his wagging tail as an emphatic, "yes."

CHAPTER 25: **THE CARE JOURNEY**

Having worked in the healthcare field for most of my career, I've witnessed firsthand how a tsunami of change in the industry has created tremendous burdens for physicians. Time constraints, the adoption of electronic medical records, intrusion of third-party payers into clinical decision-making, and the constant stress brought on by cost demands of a changing system have led many physicians to the belief that they are losing control over what's best for their patients.

Burnout has also become a major concern. Pessimism, emotional exhaustion, an inability to connect with other people, and a low sense of meaning in work have become increasingly prevalent among physicians—more so than workers in other fields, according to a study published by the Archives of Internal Medicine in 2012. Providers on the front lines of care access—general internal medicine, family practice, and emergency services—reported the highest levels of these symptoms. The accompanying stresses of burnout can lead to medical mistakes and missed diagnoses, while a lack of time to keep up with a constant flow of new medical information and advances can lead to gaps in knowledge.

Several of the doctors I've worked with believe the adoption of electronic medical record systems interfere with patient relationships and have, ironically, made their jobs more difficult. Because the EMR is currently designed more for purposes of coding and charge capture, it's not particularly intuitive for providers who focus on decision-making and diagnostics in support of their patients.

Yet another stressor is an increasing need for doctors to try to help patients find and obtain care with fewer out-of-pocket costs. Lack of health insurance has been associated with an estimated 45,000 preventable deaths per year according to the American Journal of Public Health. According to the Commonwealth Fund, in 2012, there were 31.7 million people under age 65 who were underinsured, meaning they spent a high percentage of their annual income on medical expenses. Together with the 47.3 million uninsured, this meant at least 79 million people were at risk of not being able to afford needed care. People typically fare better with employer-provided insurance, but the economic recession that began in 2007 led to millions of jobs being eliminated or replaced with part time jobs that don't provide health insurance. The result is that more of the uninsured and underinsured choose to forego seeing a doctor altogether when they are sick or hurt, but for someone with an inherited cancer syndrome or a chronic condition, the consequences of that decision can prove fatal. And for those who simply cannot avoid medical care, it can be financially devastating.

It is clear that the demands on our healthcare providers and the resulting difficulties in navigating the healthcare system are extraordinary. What then, are patients and their loved ones to do when faced with a disease or disorder such as FAP, a syndrome affecting an estimated 50,000 families in the US alone? Given the challenges facing doctors and patients struggling with the various burdens of their illness and a system that can feel as if it is working against them, it becomes necessary for those with inherited conditions like FAP to play a larger role in their care. The valuable time a doctor takes discussing diagnoses, treatment plans, and lifestyle changes with his or her patient is key to a successful patient-physician relationship, so it becomes critically important to come to appointments prepared and educated.

At the heart of diagnosing familial adenomatous polyposis and other inherited cancer syndromes is the sharing of one's family history or pedigree with your doctor. Much of the responsibility for identifying and pursuing pedigree analysis and genetic testing initially falls to primary care providers. There have been several instances throughout my adult life where I sketched out our family history of colorectal cancers and shared it with my doctors up front so they were aware of what was going on in our family. And although referral networks may be adequate for most problems, inherited cancer syndromes pose special difficulties because they can cause problems in a variety of organ systems. This requires the coordination of multiple specialists, which is why they are often referred to as "diagnostic nightmares" for physicians.

To help focus attention on the importance of family history, the Surgeon General, in conjunction with the Department of Health and Human Services and other agencies, recently launched a public health campaign. Dubbed the Surgeon General's Family Health History Initiative, it is designed to encourage all American families to learn more about their family's medical history. As part of this initiative they have developed a tool to help patients collect this information called My Family Health Portrait.

My advice, after years of dealing with and working within the system, is to be your own greatest advocate. Be well informed, be prepared, and initiate action whenever you feel it's necessary. This means keeping track of what each specialist advises and prescribes, assuring you are compliant with their recommendations, and letting any other doctors involved in your care know about it.

When families like ours keep their own thorough notes via an ongoing summary, complete with a family history and any relevant medical information, it dramatically helps facilitate the task of bringing new doctors, specialists, and genetic counselors up to speed. Patients may also want to take advantage of government agency websites such as the National Institute of Health, the National Cancer Institute, and the US Department of Health and Human Services. We learned that when diagnosed with a potentially serious medical condition, we should expect to invest extra time optimizing our knowledge of available treatment options and lifestyle changes.

Despite our horrendous experience with the oncologist assigned to my mother's case in 1997, I've found over time that he was the exception. Virtually every other encounter we've had related to the FAP syndrome and what to expect in terms of collaborative care have been with clinicians and care providers who welcomed our questions and encouraged us to stay informed about the condition. In my experience, we have everything to gain through patient and family-centered self-advocacy.

CHAPTER 26: **DEVILS LAKE**

It was a captivating autumn night, the kind that tricks most native Minnesotans into forgetting how god-awful the months to follow would be. Vibrant explosions of color, daytime temps in the 70s falling to the upper 50s at night—perfect for an evening bonfire and drinks with friends. Those fleeting fall days might be all that prevents a mass exodus from the state for those in search of more hospitable winters. Bill had built a spectacular bonfire to chase away the evening chill. In its flickering, shifting shadows, I decided to make a trip to North Dakota.

It was the fall of 2013 and Addy had started her semester at UND as a reporter for the campus newspaper, *The Dakota Student.* As luck would have it, her flair for the creative also included an ability to connect with people. Whether it was the owner of a long-standing tattoo shop located near campus or an alumnus who had donated a telescope to the University's Physics and Astrophysics departments, she had an engaging way of telling their stories. She infused humor into her articles and wasn't afraid to ask the questions that would be on the minds of her college audience. Bill and I were pleasantly surprised with this choice of a potential career path. In her mind it was a step closer to writing for *Rolling Stone* magazine.

Two weeks later, I arrived in Devils Lake from Grand Forks in the late morning following an intense fog that had blanketed the highway. White-knuckled and happy to be off the road, I settled into one of the historic archive rooms of the Lake Region Heritage Center. I sat at a table surrounded by bookshelf after bookshelf of binders containing old, yellowed newspaper clippings. I started with those from the Devils Lake Daily Journal. Most of the clippings were filed in the binders by year, so I began my search with year 1900 and looked for anything related to my mother's family. The name Regan was familiar—specifically the name Peter Regan. Born in Ireland in 1840, he crossed the Atlantic at the age of ten to join relatives in Canada. He later married a woman named Hanora Ahearn, who'd also come to North America from Ireland. They had three sons (Daniel, John, and Edward) and two daughters (Mary and Annie). They'd been homesteaders, and Peter and his older boys made their way from Canada to the Dakota Territory in 1880 during the Dakota boom years and broke sod and developed the fields. They owned and controlled some five thousand acres in what is now called Webster Township outside of Devils Lake.

As I read, it became increasingly clear that homesteading life was tough. Many Irish immigrants moved to the Dakota Territory during this time and faced backbreaking labor and natural disasters. Hardships came with each new season. Spring brought flooding. Heat and drought in the summer left streams dry and animals dead. And then there were the insect invasions. After hot, dry summers, autumn often brought tinder fires. With winter came frigid temperatures, ice, and snow.

In spite of it all, Peter Regan and his family survived and prospered. He donated forty acres of land across the road from his farm to accommodate a Catholic church and cemetery. On this land, St. Peter and Paul's Church was built by area families. The church was also known as the Regan Church. Many of my mother's relatives had been buried in the cemetery, including her great-grandmother Hanora Regan, her grandmother Mary Regan Baker, her mother Cecilia Baker Miller, her aunts Mayme Baker Garske and Kathleen Baker Connor, and her Uncle Joe Baker. As far as I was concerned, this was where the long, difficult story of our struggle with familial polyposis and the APC gene mutation began.

The cemetery would be located in Webster Township, north of Devils Lake. I pulled out a county map and found Webster. It looked to be mostly farmland and was a relatively small area geographically. I should be able to find the cemetery with little effort now that the fog had cleared.

I left the Lake Region Heritage Center and walked around downtown for a while to stretch my legs. I passed an Episcopal Church built entirely of fieldstone in the 1800s. Walking toward 4th and 5th Streets, I passed the building that had once been an old fire station back when my grandfather Reggie had been a volunteer fireman for Devils Lake. I remember my mother telling me that President Franklin Delano Roosevelt had visited Devils Lake in the 1930s, arriving by train. That, I thought, must have been a colossal event for this tiny downtown of just a few square blocks. But it was full of history and amazingly preserved buildings. Most of them had been

built between 1885 and 1914 and are now on the National
Register of Historic Places.

I stopped at Old Main Café and picked up a to-go bowl of
soup so I could continue my walk. When I'd taken in the quaint
little downtown, I got in my car destined for Webster. After a
brief stop to check in at a local hotel, I continued my search for
St. Peter and Paul's Cemetery.

I traveled due north on ND State Highway 20 toward
Starkweather, hoping I'd find the cemetery before reaching the
Canadian border. That would involve a somewhat awkward
conversation with Bill about my penchant for eschewing maps
and just figuring it out as I went along. *How hard can it be?* I
thought. *There isn't much out here.*

That, of course, assumed there would at least be signs. And
forget about GPS in that particular stretch of nowhere. You use
your gut or stop to talk to the locals. As I traveled north, people
became scarce, but there were farm fields aplenty. Yellow and
gold colored land stretched on for miles around me. Sunflowers
and wheat fields. It was breathtaking. And all too easy to take
one's eyes off the road while looking for signs. But there were
none.

Damn, I thought, *I should have contacted my mom's
cousin Mike or Mike's nephew Patrick before I drove up here.*
Karen would have had their info. As I continued driving north,
I spotted a small building to my left with a few cars out front.
Across the street was an old, boarded-up schoolhouse that I
assumed was once Webster Elementary. I was close now, for
sure. I knew it. I stopped at the building—a bar. A small neon
sign glowing bright in the window signaled it was open.

The Flyway Bar was situated on Hwy 20 next to several
houses that appeared to constitute a very tiny neighborhood.

The bar looked like one of those places where people might stop on a Friday or Saturday night to have a drink and talk about the weather. Or the new tractor. Or soybean prices. Or the game. Or maybe fishing in Devils Lake. I imagined the occasional snowmobile club might show up in winter to warm up with a cocoa or a shot of Jameson before heading back out on their sleds.

As much as I'd have liked to toss back a cold can of Iron Horse with the locals, I was anxious to talk with someone who might know where the cemetery was. I went inside. Straight ahead, a gentleman wiped off the top of the bar with a stained, white towel. The minute he saw me his face registered, *Not from around here.* I must have looked lost and was a little too excited to see him for him to assume anything else.

"Hi. I'm from Minneapolis, and I'm looking for a family cemetery," I blurted. I didn't introduce myself by name. Only later did I realize that I probably sounded rude and like I had something to hide.

He raised an eyebrow and asked, "What family might that be?"

I had to think on my feet. "Um, the Regan, or Baker, or Connor family or families?"

His demeanor changed immediately. "Oh, ya. The old Regan cemetery. It's across the street from the farmhouse, just up that road about a mile then take a right at the road grader."

"What's a road grader?" I asked.

His face said, *City girl,* but he at least managed not to roll his eyes. "A big John Deere road grader," he responded. "Ever hear of John Deere?"

Good grief, I thought. *I'm not totally clueless.*

He continued. "It's a big yellow one, parked by the road up from the cemetery and the Regan farmhouse."

I thanked him profusely. It was late in the afternoon, and I was in a rush to find it before dark. No matter what he might have thought of me, the bartender's directions were good. Look for a large yellow piece of farm equipment that isn't a tractor. I could do that. And there it was, far bigger and better than any street sign to navigate by. And of course there wouldn't be signs to the cemetery anyway; it was private.

The cemetery itself was exactly where he had described it. I pulled up to the entrance. A wrought iron sign above the locked gate told me this was the place I'd been looking for. St. Peter and Paul's Cemetery. It was small and surrounded by a wire fence, which was loose and easy to lift. I crawled under with my camera. Once inside, I immediately noticed a lovely bench to my right, facing a brick wall that told the cemetery's story and listed the surnames of the families with loved ones buried there. A large bell hung to the left of the wall.

I hadn't been in the cemetery more than two minutes when I heard the sound of a vehicle approaching and turned to see a white Suburban moving fast and spitting up a cloud of dirt from the road. I thought it would pass the entrance to the cemetery, but I was wrong. It pulled in and parked next to my car. Two men and a woman got out of the SUV. Something Bill said once in a while popped into my head: *I didn't just fall off a turnip truck.* The bartender at The Flyway must have called someone. I could only hope they were relatives because I hadn't told anyone I was coming.

The driver appeared to be not much younger than I was. He reached out his hand to greet me. While I was a bit stunned over the unexpected reception, I heard him use the name Regan.

Once the formal introductions were made, I said, "Regan? Descended from Peter Regan, who donated forty acres to build a church and this cemetery? He was my great-great-grandfather. I believe that makes us distant cousins. My great-grandmother and your great-grandfather were siblings. Nice to meet you," I said with a smile.

After those awkward first moments, their concerns about me evaporated. The woman was Mrs. Regan, and the man with them was a neighbor who also had family buried there. I told them I was looking for my grandmother's grave and apologized for sliding under the fence—I'd come a long way. It wasn't long before I was on the receiving end of a personal tour of the cemetery, complete with family histories. The Regan boys, Peter Regan's sons, lived long lives—two of them into their seventies and Edward into his eighties. It was easy to see by the dates etched in the gravestones which family line was the recipient of the mutated gene. Mary Regan Baker's.

Mr. Regan and his wife left me to my investigation of the graveyard with a promise to return to lock the gate after I'd gone. They also offered to contact my mother's cousin Mike for me. I jotted down my name and cell number down for them in the hopes that he'd have some time to visit with me before I returned to the Twin Cities the next day. I wrote a note to him in the visitor's book as well, having just discovered that he was in charge of the cemetery's oversight.

Before driving back to Devils Lake, I spent a few more moments in front of Cecilia's headstone. The grandmother I never knew. To think she'd died leaving behind a six-year-old daughter, never knowing she'd have been grandmother to eight left me feeling wistful.

I didn't look back after I closed the gates behind me. And I knew I'd never be back to that place. I'd made the physical connection I'd hoped to find. What had once been only faded black and white photographs and stories shared over dessert at the kitchen table were now real to me. I'd done what I'd come to do.

My cell phone rang a few minutes before my alarm was scheduled to go off. It was Mike on the other end, one minute giving me directions to his farm, and the next playfully chastising me for not letting him know I'd be in town. I'd last seen Mike and Ellen sometime in the early '80s at a family gathering at my parents' house. I wasn't sure I'd recognize him, but after thirty years, I figured he'd have the same problem recognizing me, so that leveled the field.

"Don't eat breakfast," he said, "Ellen will cook up something for us."

Even with actual directions to follow, I had to pay close attention to the street signs and road markers to find their farmstead. I pulled up near the garage where Mike was waiting for me beside a ladder and endless coils of lights.

I shot out of the car and gave him a colossal hug and said, "It's been a long time."

"Yes, it has," he said with a grin.

"What's with all this?" I asked him, nodding toward the ladder.

"Decorating for our last-ever Christmas light show," he said. "Too damn hard on my knees to string the lights on the barn and house these days."

For more than a quarter century, Mike and Ellen had adorned their farmyard with holiday lights and seasonal decorations. "Christmas in the Country" was a special treat for the neighbors and their families.

I heard Ellen call for us through the screen door. "Come on in! We have coffee."

"Let's go," Mike said, laying the ladder on its side and tilting his head toward the house.

We sat in the sun porch and spent some time catching up with steaming mugs of strong, black coffee before us. I mentioned the trip to Devils Lake had been more of a side trip after visiting Addy in Grand Forks, and I hadn't wanted to burden anyone with my last minute plans.

"No burden," Ellen said, smiling.

I discovered that Mike had been doing some genealogy research of his own with his nephew Patrick and had recently been in touch with my sister Karen. We talked a lot about Mike's mother (my mom's Aunt Kathleen)—how close she and Cecilia had been, and how important it had been to her to keep in touch with my mother after she'd left Devils Lake. I told Mike that I remembered many kitchen table conversations at my parents' house with Kathleen. She'd bring up her three siblings who'd died young, and with a heavy heart and tissue in hand admit that she thought there might be something "going on" in the family just as Evelyn had suggested. Her voice would trail off, and the subject would change.

Ellen returned after having disappeared into the kitchen for a bit. "We can dish up now," she said.

I smiled because I often used that term at home and Bill always poked fun at me for it. "*'Dish up?' What does that mean? Who says that*?" Now I knew where it came from.

Our meal of egg casserole, muffins, and fruit finished, the front door swung open and a tall man, maybe a few years older than me, walked in to the sunroom.

Mike stood and shook his hand and said, "Patrick, so glad you could make it." Patrick was Mike's brother Clinton's son. Clint had passed away years before.

"Of course, I see the resemblance," I teased. "I have baby pictures of you at home that my mom saved. Same smile. I'll make a point to send them to you," I promised.

Mike pushed himself away from the table and walked into the living room. From where I was sitting, I could see him digging through the drawers of a hutch, pulling out what looked to be mostly photographs. He came back to the table with a stack of pictures, most of them black and white, the subjects of the photos easily recognizable after my many years of research. There were pictures of my mom's Uncle Joe and Aunt Mayme that I'd never seen before mixed in with photos of Mike with his sister Erin, his brothers, his mom and dad, and family photos which included my grandfather, Reggie, and my mom when she was a young girl visiting in the summer months.

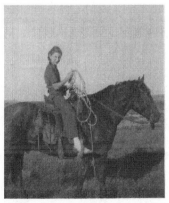

Colleen at the family farm circa 1943

Mike handed me a typed document that looked to be a letter written by my mother's Aunt Kathleen. At the top of the page were the words: I WONDER ABOUT CANCER.

My heart skipped a beat. "Do you mind if I take a few minutes to read this?" I asked.

"Of course. Take your time," he said. "I'll just go freshen up my coffee."

I WONDER ABOUT CANCER

Today I heard a friend had cancer. Ever since I can remember cancer was a hushed word in our home. Long before my time my grandmother came to this state by covered wagon from Canada, and she was only here one year before she died in 1885, and her illness was diagnosed as cancer. In the summer of 1911, my mother Mary Regan Baker was ailing with what was called summer complaint. She consulted with the doctor closest to our home, then another in a larger town, and then these two doctors consulted together. At that time there was a doctor in a small town in Minnesota who was becoming widely known for his diagnoses. It was decided my mother, accompanied by my grandfather, Peter Regan would go to see this Dr. Mayo for an examination. There a small specimen was examined with the microscope, and found to be a gland kind of colorectal cancer. Surgery was doubtful—without surgery a year or possibly more. One year later she passed away at the age of fifty-one years.

In 1924 my oldest sister 31 years old was experiencing stomach trouble. After a few trips to the hospital, surgery was decided on, the diagnosis was: cancer of the large bowel, which was removed. She lived from 2 o'clock in the afternoon until 11 o'clock the following morning.

In a couple of years my brother about 36 years old was not feeling too well in the hot weather and harvest. In October he consulted with a doctor and entered the State Veteran's Hospital. From there he underwent surgery for cancer and had a complete colostomy, and received treatment by radium following surgery. He spent about two years there, and everything known in research was used. He passed away in Hines Memorial Hospital.

In the summer of 1936, my youngest sister Cecilia was not feeling well, steadily losing weight. In August 1936 she underwent surgery, diagnosed with cancer of the colon, and her colon was removed. She passed away two weeks later.

In 1957, Cecilia's daughter was married with five small children. Her blood was low and she went for a check-up. There was a blur found on an x-ray so they decided to do exploratory surgery. She was found to have "Polyposis of the Colon." The polyps were various sizes and colors, some small and white and as yet friendly, some red ones—these were angry and some blue-grey ones—very angry and nearly malignant. She had blood transfusions before surgery; most of her colon was removed and she made a rapid recovery. Now three more healthy children later, she is a very active mother of eight children and takes part in many activities outside of her home.

Knowing all this each time I hear of cancer, I wonder just what is cancer? What change takes place in our system so we produce cancer? Why are the lumps in some members of a family malignant, and in other members of this family non-malignant? Is it a coincidence that it occurred at the same age and at the same place in the body of my two sisters? Why did it occur in my sisters, one older and one younger, and miss me so far? Why did doctors know and recognize cancer in 1885, and the same in 1968, and still no shot for cancer. Diabetes if discovered is controlled. T.B. is now arrested, but no program for cancer. It is the greatest killer of children, but is there a school check-up? Surgery or cutting it out and we keep producing it, who wins? Is it an animal to man related disease? We need new warning signals, to me, fatigue, loss of appetite, sleeplessness and tension, to name a few.

During my lifetime our country has financed two World Wars, and well into a third. What about an all out war on Cancer? The weapons, the education, and research.

New business in 1968 is for a landing on the moon next year. Old unfinished business here in this world, a research war on cancer speeded up.

When I hear of cancer these and many more questions come across my mind.

Kathleen Ann Connor

I estimated Kathleen's letter had been written in 1968, a year before Markie died. Forty-five years later, sitting in her family home reading her letter, her words conveyed the heartbreak of generations. I slowly traced her name on the fragile final page of her letter with a finger, as if trying to send her a message that, at last, I had the answers. I wished I could take her hand, look into her soft, blue-gray eyes and tell her all I'd learned.

Mike had returned from the kitchen and was watching me intently. I cleared my throat and changed the subject to keep the tears at bay.

"Out of curiosity, do you know how my mom ended up with William and Adele as her guardians? Her father was still alive and remarried within a few years. How did that come about?" I knew that in those days, what was "in the best interest of the child" often outweighed even the parents' rights.

"I don't honestly know for sure," said Mike. "Aunt Adele and my mom had a lot of influence over that decision. That I do know."

"It probably didn't help that Reggie had a reputation as a ladies' man, and he and Olive liked to tip a few back. And he was a Protestant," I said.

Patrick laughed, "That last one would have been a deal breaker."

I laughed with him. "Reggie never really had a chance. That ended up being a good thing, I think."

"By the way," Mike continued, "What happened to Adele. You know, after William divorced her?"

I sat up straighter in my chair, glad to be given a chance to speak on behalf of Auntie Del. "She had a great life with us. She could have washed her hands of our family but didn't. She was as much a grandmother to my brothers and sisters and I as anyone."

That prompted Mike to bring the conversation around to my family. He and Patrick and Ellen listened intently to the family health history, and to my account of what had happened over the previous seven years. When I described how the gene we'd inherited through the Regan-Baker line had wreaked havoc in our family and what we'd learned about the polyposis syndrome, the conversation became subdued. In describing Eric and Andrea's deaths, I needed a distraction because I had a difficult time looking them in the eye. I held my white dinner napkin down on the table with my left thumb and forefinger and smoothed it out from the center to the corners with my right hand, worrying out the wrinkles and imperfections.

"My mom used to do that!" Mike exclaimed. "Whenever she was fretting or anxious she'd do exactly what you're doing with her napkin or handkerchief. Good grief, how weird is that? Remember Pat?"

Patrick smiled. "Must be genetic," he said.

I smiled too. Then Mike asked if I'd like to take a drive out to the Baker farmstead, where my mother was born.

"I'd *love* that," I said.

CHAPTER 27: OUT CAME THE SUN

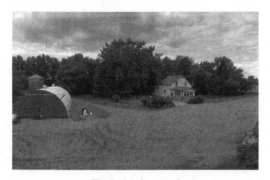

The Baker farmstead

When I first saw the house on the Baker farmstead as we drove onto the property, it didn't look particularly familiar. It was painted a light yellow, but in the black and white photos—now carefully stored in a closet at my home—it was just a large, white house. And the porch windows were different.

As I parked my car, I spotted a woman standing near a large garden, cradling an armload of dirt-riddled squash. She approached us as we walked toward her and said, "Hi, I'm Brigit, Patrick's sister. You must be Laura."

I had to keep myself from reaching out to touch her hair. It was the exact striking shade of auburn my mother and Addy had been blessed with. Mike, Ellen, and Patrick remained standing on the grass near the garden, admiring the bounty of squash and discussing how to finish up some work on the outbuildings before winter came.

Brigit placed the squash on the ground, grabbed my arm, and steered me toward the house. "A quick tour," she said.

Inside, the furnishings were comfortable but sparse. I couldn't tell if anyone was living there. In the kitchen was a table and chairs that had been in the family for over a hundred years. Framed photographs of family milestones lined the staircase wall—new babies, graduations, weddings, and anniversary celebrations. I could have been standing in my own house, or in the house on Shryer Avenue in Roseville.

After we exchanged pleasantries and got to know one another a little bit, the conversation turned to the reason for my visit. As a healthcare worker and organic farmer, Brigit was fascinated by what I'd learned about FAP.

I told her about the gene mutation and how it had been passed down through Cecilia's bloodline and its life-altering consequences for the family. During our conversation, I learned that she and I were the same age—had I come to the farm as a kid, the two of us would have definitely been fast friends. Keeping an eye on the time, Brigit and I walked back outside to join the group. I walked over to the garden for a last look around. To be standing on the land where my mother was born and where her mother had lived as young girl was overwhelming.

Brigit stepped to where I was standing and offered me several large buttercup and a few acorn squash. "For Thanksgiving dinner," she said. "They keep well."

Ah yes, I realized, *Thanksgiving is next month. I'll have to think about our plans for this year on the drive home.* That was my favorite part of going solo on a road trip—the quiet time to reflect and think.

"It was nice seeing you," Mike said as he walked me to my car.

"You as well," I replied. "And please stay off those ladders—it makes me nervous!" I stopped and gave him another hug. "It's been a wonderful couple of days. Thank you so much for showing me around and filling me in on the family history. And I'm sorry we drifted as we did; my side of the family fell off an emotional cliff there for a while. But we're slowly coming back."

"We understand," Patrick said. "Come on back up anytime. We can take Bill out fishing on Devils Lake."

As I sat down in the front seat of my car, I turned back to them. "My mother so loved it here. And all of you." I put the key in the ignition and added, "And Bill would relish fishing Devils Lake—as long as it's not ice fishing." I started up the car, and waved. As I drove away, I watched them growing smaller in my rearview mirror until they faded from view. Gone from my sight, perhaps, but just as large now as when I left them.

As it had been decided by her Aunt Kathleen and Uncle William, my mother Colleen, who'd inherited the FAP gene from her dead mother, was taken from Devils Lake to be raised by relatives. She eventually settled in St. Paul, later falling in love and marrying a charming young man with an intellectually curious mother who convinced her to see the best doctors and surgeons when it mattered most. Had my mother stayed in North Dakota, who knows what kind of life she might have had, or how long that life might have been. The key to her survival in the face of that as yet undiagnosed condition was, ironically, to leave family behind in North Dakota. Over time, her ties back to the farm may have frayed but they'd never fractured.

Twelve years is but a blink of an eye in a family's history—the time it took for her to go from being a motherless child to becoming a mother herself. This inherited syndrome does not necessarily take a straight path from A to B. When you are born can make a difference. Where you live can make a difference. Your doctor's knowledge, and where you receive treatment can make a difference. And sometimes, despite following all the rules and having access to the best medical care in the world, none of those differences matter. That has been the most difficult lesson for me in this more than 100-year journey for my family.

I smiled to myself as I passed beneath the sign for Interstate 94 East towards Minneapolis and St. Paul while recalling something Alex had said to me during one of our all-too-infrequent phone conversations during his surgery internship year at Northwestern. He'd called me on a Saturday afternoon after the topic of the physician Grand Rounds he'd attended that day was Familial Adenomatous Polyposis.

"Don't forget about the good genes we inherited, Mom," he said. "There are a lot of them. And be sure to stay compliant with your thyroid medication like we talked about, okay?"

My thoughts traveled to the Serenity Prayer. Once taped to my mother's refrigerator, it is now taped to mine, right next to a James Watson quote from a 1999 Time magazine article entitled, "All for the Good: Why Genetic Engineering Must Soldier On." It states, "Moving forward will not be for the faint of heart. But if the next century witnesses failure, let it be because our science is not yet up for the job, not because we don't have the courage to make less random the sometimes most unfair courses of human evolution." Since then, scientists and geneticists have followed the human genome project into worlds we could only imagine a decade ago. Among these advances are gene editing technologies that can alter, delete, or change the DNA of living things. It's a thorny subject for some, leading to conversations about "designer babies" and playing God. But for those who have suffered the effects of an inherited disease such as FAP, the questions become very personal. If you knew your child had a chance of inheriting a catastrophic genetic disorder, would you not want to do everything in your power to protect them from it?

Of my grandmother Cecilia's generation, 60 percent had the mutation. Then, of my parents' eight children, 62 percent were carriers of the mutated gene. Thirty-three percent of my parents' twenty-one grandchildren then inherited FAP, and of their great-grandchildren, 10 percent are carriers. Based upon living great-grandchildren and those who may be born in the future to parents who did not inherit the APC mutation, we may finally be able to bring this lineage of familial polyposis to an end.

The sum of all of our cells defines us far more than a microscopic stretch of junk on chromosome 5. We have never been defined by the faults in our genes. We are farmers, carpenters, business people, social workers, police officers, doctors, and nurses. We are mothers and fathers and grandparents. Syndromes such as FAP, Lynch Syndrome, BRCA I and II, and other inherited cancer syndromes often impact people in the prime of their lives—their most productive years. This, more than any other reason, makes me hopeful that our pursuit of knowledge and understanding will eventually bring them to an end. Or that we'll, as James Watson said, "have the courage to make them less random."

The universal corrections, both microscopic and astronomical, the ravaging and the radiant, will happen regardless. Familial Adenomatous Polyposis (FAP) is no longer the devastating, terminal disease it was to my family at the turn of the 20th century. Today, medical advancements allow for more timely and precise surveillance and treatments. My mother's grandchildren and great-grandchildren are blessed to live at a time when polyposis syndrome is considered a manageable disease with elevated risks as opposed to an inevitable early cancer. And we are currently on the cusp of genetic understanding that may well allow for such marvels as repairing the APC gene mutation forever.

If this often-painful journey has taught me anything, it's that loss reminds us of those things that are truly valuable—our relationships, family, health, and a faith in something larger than ourselves. I learned, too, that part of building resilience sometimes means letting go—using knowledge as a form of preparedness, while understanding it cannot always provide the answers we're looking for. And I've discovered that being kind to oneself and practicing gratefulness are critical parts of the healing process.

I'm especially grateful for those who have been there for us over the years and always seemed to know just what to say to help ease the anguish—if even for a moment. And for the gentle kindness of strangers. And for my family—how extraordinary that something so devastating also connected us as a force to be reckoned with. Through all of my heartache, I never once felt alone.

I switched lanes while keeping one eye on the road and the other on the speedometer. My thoughts drifted toward Thanksgiving. Would Addy be able to help me pull off a full-course homemade Thanksgiving dinner? I bet she would. And accompanying the turkey this year would be organically grown squash from a family farm. *Our* family farm.

Dusk was falling, and as I drove through Alexandria I looked out to my right at a slight dip in the road. It was almost as if someone had tapped me on the shoulder. The deep green grass of the rural landscape and the intense orange and red hues of the leaves on the treetops all met at the horizon line of the setting sun in the western sky. It was a luminous burst of brilliant, natural beauty; I may never again see its equal. It was another truly lived moment. I was once again overwhelmed by gratitude.

I couldn't wait to be back home.

AFTERWORD by Alexander J. Kieger, MD

My interest in medicine grew from an early age, largely influenced through shared hardships of many extended family members living with a rare inherited cancer syndrome, Familial Adenomatous Polyposis. Needless to say, I am deeply fulfilled by their continued encouragement and the enduring value of their perspectives as both patients and loved ones. That continuous circle of encouragement has been a source of strength, even at our most crushing moments as a family.

I had decided in March of 2007 to enter an entrepreneur competition aimed to challenge students to show creativity and innovation in solving health care related problems. I was a junior at the time. Despite my mind being a tangle of mental notes and last minute changes, I never let myself waver from the road ahead. The previous few days had been a blur, as I had let a good night's sleep repeatedly escape me in order to perfect my presentation. Behind the wheel of my car, my thoughts turned to what had inspired me to enter this contest. It was for the same reason I studied basic sciences as an undergraduate, and was pursuing a career in medicine. In that moment, with my goals and accomplishments a small monument against prior adversity, I was replete with confidence and hope. But just as the world seemed wonderful and justified, my cell phone rang. On the other line was my mother's voice. In a despondent tone all too familiar to me, she explained that my thirty-one-year-old cousin Andrea had suddenly died of complications of her brain tumor. The news was almost too much to bear. The emotional sores from my uncle Eric's passing, under similar circumstances just months earlier, were still fresh. Mixed with my immediate grief and feelings of being mocked by the world, I felt a tiny reassurance that I had chosen the right direction. After ending a brief but heartfelt conversation with my mother, I wiped the tears from my eyes, quieted my mind, and once again focused on the long road ahead.

I am proud that most of the foundational lessons I learned about being a doctor were from my own family. Modern medicine is a mountain of human accomplishments, and forthcoming advancements in disease treatment and early detection are a constant source of optimism. And while digital technology rapidly transforms the healthcare experience for patients and providers, it must maintain patient engagement and education as a high priority in its engineering. One important reason is for patients to ensure they stay on track with appointments and screening exams, especially as they move through different care networks and doctors during their lifetime. In part, my mother's beautifully thoughtful storytelling explores our own experience navigating the healthcare system with a familial cancer syndrome, and illustrates pivotal instances when gaps in knowledge and expert guidance gave rise to moments of tragedy.

Similar missteps still occur today, even in our modern technology-driven healthcare system. There is no denying that electronic health records greatly improve medical practice, allowing doctors to better track changes in health over time, reduce medication errors, notify patients who are due for preventive visits and screenings, and collaborate with other providers. However, electronic systems can also be a hindrance to quality of care on a broader level, where compatibility issues often create barriers to exchanging and using information between different hospital networks. A study by The Office of the National Coordinator for Health Information Technology (a division of the U.S. Department of Health and Human Services) found that in 2015, only 38 percent of U.S. non-federal acute care hospitals are using or integrating records from sources outside their own health network.[1]

Any American, regardless of genetic makeup, can be at greater risk for a too-late diagnosis or incorrect care plan if their electronic health records are unusable when they re-establish care. Changing doctors and healthcare systems due to circumstances related to job loss or an equally catastrophic life event are unfortunately a common experience for American families. Large stacks of scanned paper documents are an unsatisfactory substitute—often time-consuming to read in detail, and unfamiliar formatting can lead to important information being overlooked. This can be mitigated when

---

[1] https://dashboard.healthit.gov/evaluations/data-briefs/non-federal-acute-care-hospital-interoperability-2015.php#

patients are knowledgeable about their own health and prior care plans, and make sure to cover important details during the history and physical exam. Patients are urged to keep good personal medical records including information related to family history. Patients also benefit greatly from staying within a center of excellence for particular disease, and need to be active in making sure they are getting care at the right place.

Even so, a good patient-provider relationship is the foundation that cannot be replaced. Patients can be unfamiliar with or uncomfortable using patient portals, and care networks need to make sure that these interfaces are tailored to patient education and reading level. Care networks also need to be held accountable when they are unable to send, receive and use electronic health records from an outside source, which Congress recently declared a national objective.[2]

We are entering a time in history where advancements in the understanding of genetics and cancer are accelerating beyond even what I could comprehend as an undergraduate student participating in a competition to address healthcare related problems. While seemingly beyond imagination as to where nanotechnology, immunology, advanced imaging and genomics will take us, the need for thoughtful conversation between doctor and patient is still the greatest diagnostic and therapeutic tool of all.

Our hope is that readers and their families who read our story will be inspired to proactively engage with their providers,

---

[2] Medicare Access and CHIP Reauthorization Act of 2015 (MACRA), Congress declared it a national objective to achieve widespread exchange of health information through interoperable certified electronic health record (EHR) technology nationwide by December 31, 2018 (1)

become informed healthcare consumers, take charge of their health information empowering them to overcome barriers to quality care, and most of all to advocate tirelessly on behalf of themselves and their loved ones.

Alexander J. Kieger, MD
Resident, Radiology
Johns Hopkins
Baltimore, Maryland

NOTES

Summer's Complaint is the culmination of many years of research. Sources include innumerable conversations and interviews with family members, friends, co-workers, and healthcare providers as well as review of historical, legal, and medical documents and records that are in the author's possession. Additional sources include newspaper articles and related materials within the public domain, including birth and death records. Source material beyond the aforementioned are listed by chapter and page below. Every effort has been made to attribute credit where it is due.

Images and Words

p15: "...years later made it into the local newspaper as part of the story...": Bachmeier, Cam. "Yesteryears: Photos Bring Back Many Memories." *Grand Forks Herald,* October 1, 2005. Photo: "The Fabulous Baker Girls."

Find the Families

p55: "It's possible that my grandmother may have read about Dr. Cuthbert Dukes...": St. Mark's Academic Institute. "History of the Registry."
http://www.stmarksacademicinstitute.org.uk/specialities/medicine/polyposis-registry/

p56: "Dukes would publish his seminal report..." Bülow, Steffen, Terri Berk, Kay Neale. "The History of Familial Adenomatous Polyposis." *Familial Cancer* no. 5 (2006): 213-220 doi: 10.1007/s10689-005-5854-0 p56: "At a presentation of his work at the Mayo Clinic…" Dukes, Cuthbert. Mayo Foundation Lecture presented on 10/24/58. Published in *Diseases of the Colon and Rectum* 1, no. 6 (Nov/Dec 1958): 413-423

pp56-57: "You are old, Father William, the young surgeon said…" Bülow, Steffen, Terri Berk, Kay Neale. "The History of Familial Adenomatous Polyposis." *Familial Cancer* no. 5 (2006): 213-220 doi: 10.1007/s10689-005-5854-0

p57: "…read a one-page paper describing the findings of…": Watson, James and Francis Crick. "A Structure for Deoxyribose Nucleic Acid." *Nature* 171 (1953): 737-738.

p57: "Even after the discovery of the double helix…": National Institutes of Health, National Human Genome Research Institute. "Genetic Timeline." https://www.genome.gov/pages/education/genetictimeline.pdf

pp57-58: "As Eldon J. Gardner, an early researcher…" Gardner, Eldon J., "Genetics of Cancer and Other Abnormal Growths" (1954). *USU Faculty Honor Lectures.* Paper 27. http://digitalcommons.usu.edu/honor_lectures/27

p58: "As an Internal Medicine resident at the University of Nebraska…": Creighton University School of Medicine website Welcome Page. "Chair of Preventative Medicine: Henry Lynch, MD." http://medschool.creighton.edu/centers/hcc/welcome/

p58: "Dr. Lynch postulated that some of these cancers might have hereditary origins": Cantor, David. "The Frustration of Families: Henry Lynch, Heredity, and Cancer Control, 1962-1975." *Cambridge Journals of Medical History* 50, no. 3 (July 2006): 279-302. doi: 10.1017/S0025727300009996.

Working the Plan

p74: "Gregor Mendel was an Australian monk...": National Institutes of Health, National Human Genome Research Institute. "Talking Glossary of Genetic Terms: Mendelian Inheritance." https://www.genome.gov/glossary/

p74: "Gregor Mendel was an Australian monk...": Applewhite, Ashton, Jay Brown, and Joan Greco. *Our Genes/Our Choices.* TV Documentary. Directed by Mark Ganguzza and Barbara Margolis. Fred Friendly Seminars, Thirteen/WNET, 2003.

p77: "Remarkably, as reported in the 1980 Journal of Opthamology..." (from the Minneapolis evening paper): Blair, Norman P. and Clement L. Trempe. "Hypertrophy of the Retinal Pigment Epithelium Associated with Gardner's Syndrome." *American Journal of Ophthalmology* 90, no. 5 (November 1980): 661-63, 665-67. doi: 10.1016/S0002-9394(14)75133-5.

Bench Strength

p95: "Dr. Cuthbert Dukes' laboratory assistant, H.J.R. Bussey...": St. Mark's Academic Institute. "History of the Registry." http://www.stmarksacademicinstitute.org.uk/specialities/medicine/polyposis-registry/

p95: "His thesis, Familial Polyposis Coli...": Bussey, H.J.R. *Familial Polyposis Coli: Family Studies, Histopathology, Differential Diagnosis, and Results of Treatment.* (Baltimore: Johns Hopkins University Press, 1975).

pp95-96: "In 1977, Frederick Sanger developed...": Genome: Unlocking Life's Code website, "Timeline." https://unlockinglifescode.org/timeline/11

p96: "In 1986, a research team from the U.S. published a paper...": Arney, Kat. "Chasing Down the APC Bowel Cancer Gene." Cancer Research UK website, November 29, 2011. http://scienceblog.cancerresearchuk.org/2011/11/29/high-impact-science-chasing-down-the-apc-bowel-cancer-gene/

p96: "Later that same year, in October of 1986, the Minneapolis Star Tribune...": Newhouse News Service. "Jaw, Eye May Give Clues to Colon-Cancer Risk." *Minneapolis Star Tribune,* October 10, 1986.

Finally, a Test

p122: "While we were relatively sure by then that I wasn't a carrier...": American Medical Association. "Colorectal Cancer Fact Sheet: Understand the Basics of Genetic Testing for Hereditary Colorectal Cancer." (Updated February 2012).

p123: "It wasn't until the 1980s that the field of genetic counseling began to grow rapidly...": New York State Genetic Counseling Information Resource website. "History of Genetic Counseling." http://www.nysgeneticcounselors.org/history.php

p127: "...busyness...serves the same psychological role that it always has...": Burkeman, Oliver. "Why Time Management is Ruining Our Lives." *The Guardian,* December 22, 2016.

Beloved Brother

p143: "...how to make an appointment at Memorial Sloan-Kettering...": Memorial Sloan-Kettering Cancer Center. https://www.mskcc.org

p143: "...how a physician can make a referral to MD Anderson...": MD Anderson Cancer Center—Physician Referral Resources. https://www.mdanderson.org/for-physicians/refer-a-patient.html

p144: "Diagnosed at an advanced stage, as Eric's cancer was...": National Cancer Institute. (General information related to gastric cancer) http://www.cancer.gov

p146: "I remember watching the slideshow, *The Interview with God*...": http://www.theinterviewwithgod.com Gregory Writer, Angel Network LLC, 2008

Down Came the Rain

A number of websites and resources were accessed between January of 2006 and May of 2007 related to my Internet searches following the cancer diagnoses of my brother and niece. Included are:

Lynch, Henry T. and Thomas C. Smyrk. "Classification of Familial Adenomatous Polyposis: A Diagnostic Nightmare." *American Journal of Human Genetics* 62 (1998): 1288-9. doi: 10.1086/301890.

Lynch, Henry T., Trudy G. Shaw, and Jane F. Lynch. "Inherited Predisposition to Cancer: A Historical Overview." *American Journal of Medical Genetics Part C: Seminars in Medical Genetics* 129C, no. 1 (July 2004): 5-22. doi: 10.1002/ajmg.c.30026.

Jasperson, Kory W., Swati G. Patel, and Dennis J. Ahnen. "APC-Associated Polyposis Conditions." *Gene Reviews* (December 18, 1998, last updated, February 2, 2017). https://www.ncbi.nlm.nih.gov/books/NBK1345/

PDQ® Adult Treatment Editorial Board. PDQ Gastric Cancer Treatment. Bethesda, MD: National Cancer Institute. Updated 07/01/2016. Available at: https://www.cancer.gov/types/stomach/patient/stomach-treatment-pdq PMID: 26389328

Iida, M., T. Yao, H. Itoh, H. Watanabe, T. Matsui, A. Iwashita, and M. Fujishima "Natural History of Gastric Adenomas in Patients with Familial Adenomatous Coli/Gardners' Syndrome." *Cancer* 61, no. 3 (February 1, 1988): 605-11. PMID: 338026.

Bulow, S, J Bjork, IJ Christensen, O Fausa, H Järvinen, F Moesgaard, and HFA Vasen. "Duodenal Adenomatosis in Familial Adenomatous Polyposis." *Gut* 53, no. 3 (March 2004): 381-6. doi: 10.1136/gut.2003.027771.

Kadmon, Martina, A. Tandara, and C. Herfarth. "Duodenal Adenomatosis in Familial Adenomatous Polyposis Coli. A Review of the Literature and Results from the Heidelberg Polyposis Register." *International Journal of Colorectal Disease* 16, no. 2 (April 2001): 63-75. PMID: 11355321.

Talamini, Mark A., Robert C. Moesinger, Herny A. Pitt, Taylor A. Sohn, Ralph H. Hruban, Keith D. Lillemoe, Charles J. Yeo, and John L. Cameron. "Adenocarcinoma of the Ampulla of Vater. A 28-Year Experience." *Annals of Surgery* 225, no. 5 (May 1997): 590-600.

Expression

p155: "...mutations can vary in their expressivity...": De Rosa, Martina, Maria I. Scarano, Luigi Panariello, Gemma Morelli, Gabrielle Riegler, Giovanni B. Rossi, Alfonso Tempesta, et al. "The Mutation Spectrum of the APC Gene in FAP Patients from Southern Italy: Detection of Known and Four Novel Mutations." *Human Mutation, Mutation in Brief* #622 (2003). doi: 10.1002/humu.9151.

p155: "...mutations can vary in their expressivity...": Crabtree, M. D., P. M. Tomlinson, S. V. Hodgson, K. Neale, R. K. S. Phillips, and R. S. Houlston. "Exploring Variation in Familial Adenomatous Polyposis: Relationship Between Genotype and Phenotype and Evidence for Modifier Genes." *Gut* 51, no. 3 (September 2002): 420-3. doi: 10.1136/gut.51.3.420.

p156: "There are nineteen alleles associated with our mutation address, Codon 1068.": Friedl, Waltraut and Stefan Aretz. "Familial Adenomatous Polyposis: Experience from a Study of 1164 Unrelated German Polyposis Patients." *Hereditary Cancer in Clinical Practice* 3, no. 3 (September 2005): 95-114. doi: 10.1186/1897-4287-3-3-95.

Freefall

p173: "...it can take as many as seventeen years for basic research to move...": Morris, Zoe Slote, Steven Wooding, Jonathan Grant. "The Answer is 17 Years, What is the Question: Understanding Time Lags in Translational Research." *Journal of the Royal Society of Medicine* 104, no. 12 (December 2011): 510-520. doi: 10.1258/jrsm.2011.110180.

Era of the Genome

p174: "In 1990, the National Institute of Health and the Department of Energy...": National Institutes of Health. "Human Genome Project Fact Sheet." https://report.nih.gov/NIHfactsheets/ViewFactSheet.aspx?csid=45

p174: "In 1990, the National Institute of Health and the Department of Energy...": National Institutes of Health, National Human Genome Research Institute. "Genetic Timeline." https://www.genome.gov/pages/education/genetictimeline.pdf

p174: "In 1990, the National Institute of Health and the Department of Energy...": National Institutes of Health, National Human Genome Research Institute. "Genetics: The Future of Medicine." https://www.genome.gov/pages/educationkit/images/nhgri.pdf

p174: "...tumor suppressor gene, which normally produces a protein...": Peel, Nick. "Turning Off Bowel Cancer—as easy as APC?" Cancer Research UK website, June 18, 2015. http://scienceblog.cancerresearchuk.org/2015/06/18/turning-off-bowel-cancer-as-easy-as-apc/

p175: "...two teams from the U.S., one from Utah and another from Baltimore...": (Johns Hopkins Team) Kinzler, K. W., M. C. Nilbert, L. K. Su, B. Vogelstein , T. M. Bryan, D. B. Levy, K. J. Smith, A. C. Preisinger, P. Hedge, D. McKechnie, et al. "Identification of FAP Locus Genes from Chromosome 5q21." *Science* 253, no. 5020 (August 9, 1991): 661-5.

p175: "...two teams from the U.S., one from Utah and another from Baltimore...": (Utah team) Groden, J., A. Thliveris, W. Samowitz, M. Carlson, L. Gelbert, H. Albertsen, G. Joslyn, J. Stevens, L. Spiro, M. Robertson, et al. "Identification and Characterization of the Familial Adenomatous Polyposis Coli Gene." *Cell* 66, no. 3 (August 9, 1991): 589-600.

p175: "That same day, August 9, 1991...": Angier, Natalie. "Doctors Link Gene to Colon Cancer." *New York Times*, August 9, 1991

p176: "Nobel Laureate James D. Watson stated..." National Institutes of Health, National Human Genome Research Institute. "International Consortium Completes Human Genome Project." April 14, 2003. https://www.genome.gov/11006929/

Johns Hopkins Bound

p189: "Over the years, we'd come to understand the difficulties and challenges...": Worthen, Hilary G. "Inherited Cancer and the Primary Care Physician: Barriers and Strategies." *Cancer* 86, no. 11 supplemental (December 1999): 2583-8.

The Care Journey

p195: "...according to a study published...": The Physicians Foundation. "A Survey of America's Physicians: Practice Patterns and Perspectives. An Examination of the Professional Morale, Practice Patterns, Career Plans, and Healthcare Perspectives of Today's Physicians, Aggregated by Age, Gender, Primary Care/Specialists, and Practice Owners/Employees." Survey conducted by Merritt Hawkins, September 2012. http://www.physiciansfoundation.org/uploads/default/ Physicians_Foundation_2012_Biennial_Survey.pdf p195: "Burnout has also become a major concern.": Shanafelt, Tait D, Sonja Boone, and Litjen Tan, et al. "Burnout and Satisfaction With Work-Life Balance Among US Physicians Relative to the General US Population." *Archives of Internal Medicine*. 172, no. 18 (October 8, 2012): 1377-85. doi: 10.1001/archinternmed.2012.3199.

p195: "Burnout has also become a major concern.": Snowbeck, Christopher. "Doctors Battling Crisis of Burnout." *Minneapolis Star Tribune*, August 7, 2016.

p196: "According to the Commonwealth Fund...": Schoen, Cathy, Susan L. Hayes, Sara R. Collins, Jacob A. Lippa, and David C. Radley. "America's Underinsured: A State-by-State Look at Health Insurance Affordability Prior to the New Coverage Expansions." *The Commonwealth Fund*, March 2014.

p196: "...there were 31.7 million people under age 65 who were underinsured...": Chokshi, Niraj. "Historians Take Note: What America Looked Like Before Obamacare." *Washington Post*, March 26, 2014.

pp197-198: "...the Surgeon General, in conjunction with the Department of Health...": U.S. Department of Heath and Human Services. "About the Surgeon General's Family Health History Initiative." http://www.hhs.gov/programs/prevention-and-wellness/family-health-history/about-family-health-history/index.html

Devils Lake

pp200-201: "Hardships came with each new season...": Bradsher, Greg. "How the West Was Settled. The 150-Year-Old Homestead Act Lured Americans Looking for a New Life and New Opportunities." *Prologue Magazine* (Winter 2012): 27-35.

Out Came the Sun

p218: "Moving forward will not be for the faint of heart...":
Watson, James. "All for the Good: Why Genetic Engineering
Must Soldier On." *Time* 153, no. 1 (January 11, 1999): 91

**General sources accessed and reviewed related to FAP
throughout my writing:**

McKusick, Victor A and Cassandra L. Kniffin, et al. "Familial
Adenomatous Polyposis 1; FAP1." *Online Mandelian
Inheritance in Man* (June 1986)
http://omim.org/entry/175100

Half, Elizabeth, Dani Bercovich, and Paul Rozen. "Familial
Adenomatous Polyposis." *Orphanet Journal of Rare Diseases*
4, no. 22 (October 2009) doi: 10.1186/1750-1172-4-22

Syngal, Sapna, Randall E. Brand, James M. Church, Francis M.
Giardiello, Heather L. Hampel, and Randall W. Burt. "ACG
Clinical Guideline: Genetic Testing and Management of
Hereditary Gastrointestinal Cancer Syndromes." *American
Journal Gastroenterology* 110 (February 2015): 233-62. doi
10.1038/ajg.2014.435.

National Institutes of Health, U.S. National Library of
Medicine. "Your Guide to Understanding Genetic Conditions."
Genetics Home Reference (October 2013)
https://ghr.nlm.nih.gov/condition/familial-adenomatous-
polyposis

National Institute of Health (NIH): https://www.nih.gov/

U.S. National Library of Medicine: http://www.nlm.nih.gov

National Cancer Institute: https://www.cancer.gov

The Cancer Genome Atlas (TCGA):
https://cancergenome.nih.gov

Cancer Moonshot: https://www.cancer.gov/research/key-initiatives/moonshot-cancer-initiative

The Genomic Data Commons (GDC): https://gdc.cancer.gov

National Human Genome Research Institute:
https://www.genome.gov/

GeneReviews: https://www.ncbi.nlm.nih.gov/books/NBK1116/

NORD: National Organization for Rare Disorders:
https://rarediseases.org/rare-diseases/familial-adenomatous-polyposis/

U.S. National Library of Medicine: http://www.nlm.nih.gov

RESOURCES

General Resources

American Cancer Society:
https://www.cancer.org/

American Society of Human Genetics (ASHG):
https://www.ashg.org

Cancer Action Network (American Cancer Society):
https://acscan.org/

Cancer Moonshot:
https://www.cancer.gov/research/key-initiatives/moonshot-cancer-initiative

GeneReviews:
https://www.ncbi.nlm.nih.gov/books/NBK1116/

Genetics Home Reference—Familial Adenomatous Polyposis:
(Excellent site for information on FAP complete with downloadable PDFs and other resources for patients and their families.)
https://ghr.nlm.nih.gov/condition/familial-adenomatous-polyposis

The Genomic Data Commons (GDC):
https://gdc.cancer.gov

National Cancer Institute:
https://www.cancer.gov

National Cancer Institute: Colorectal Cancer:
https://www.cancer.gov/types/colorectal

National Cancer Institute: Genetics of Colorectal Cancer:
https://www.cancer.gov/types/colorectal/hp/colorectal-genetics-pdq

National Human Genome Research Institute:
https://www.genome.gov/

National Human Genome Research Institute: Learning About
Colon Cancer:
https://www.genome.gov/10000466/

National Institute of Diabetes and Digestive and Kidney
Diseases—Colon Polyps:
https://www.niddk.nih.gov/health-information/digestive-diseases/colon-polyps

National Institute of Health (NIH):
https://www.nih.gov/

Office of Disease Prevention and Health Promotion:
https://health.gov

PubMed (comprises more than 26 million citations for
biomedical literature from MEDLINE, life science journals, and
online books):
https://www.ncbi.nlm.nih.gov/pubmed

Surgeon General's My Family Health Portrait:
https://familyhistory.hhs.gov/FHH/html/index.html

The Cancer Genome Atlas (TCGA):
https://cancergenome.nih.gov

U.S. National Library of Medicine:
http://www.nlm.nih.gov

Educational Resources

American Cancer Society, Colon and Rectum Cancer:
https://www.cancer.org/cancer/colon-rectal-cancer.html

CDC: Colorectal (Colon) Cancer:
https://www.cdc.gov/cancer/colorectal/

Creighton University School of Medicine—Hereditary Cancer
Center:
http://medschool.creighton.edu/centers/hcc/

Disease InfoSearch—Attenuated Familial Adenomatous
Polyposis (AFAP):
http://www.diseaseinfosearch.org/Attenuated+Familial+
Adenomatous+Polyposis+%28AFAP%29/661

Disease InfoSearch—Familial Adenomatous Polyposis (FAP):
http://www.diseaseinfosearch.org/Familial+Adenomatous+
Polyposis+%28FAP%29/2722

Gene Reviews—APC-Associated Polyposis Conditions:
https://www.ncbi.nlm.nih.gov/books/NBK1345

Gene Reviews—MUTYH-Associated Polyposis:
https://www.ncbi.nlm.nih.gov/books/NBK107219

Genetic Science Learning Center, University of Utah:
http://learn.genetics.utah.edu/content/disorders/multifactorial/

Johns Hopkins Cancer Risk Assessment Program:
http://www.hopkinsmedicine.org/gastroenterology_
hepatology/clinical_services/colon_cancer_risk_assessment_
clinic.html

MalaCards—adenomatous polyposis coli:
http://www.malacards.org/card/adenomatous_polyposis_coli

Mount Sinai Hospital Kid's Corner—FAP & You:
http://www.zanecohencentre.com/gi-cancers/fgicr/kids-
korner/fap-a-you

My46 Trait Profile—Familial Adenomatous Polyposis:
https://www.my46.org/trait-document?trait=Familial
adenomatous polyposis&type=profile

My46 Trait Profile—MUTYH-Associated Polyposis:
https://www.my46.org/trait-document?trait=MUTYH-
Associated Polyposis&type=profile

National Organization for Rare Disorders (NORD):
https://rarediseases.org/rare-diseases/familial-adenomatous-
polyposis/

Orphanet—Familial adenomatous polyposis:
http://www.orpha.net/consor/cgi-bin/OC_Exp.php?Lng=EN&
Expert=733

Patient Support and Advocacy Resources

Agency for Healthcare Research and Quality (AHRQ):
https://www.cdc.gov/genomics/famhistory/

American Society of Colon and Rectal Surgeons—Hereditary
Colorectal Cancer Registries:
https://www.fascrs.org/hereditary-colorectal-cancer-registries

ClinicalTrials.gov:
https://clinicaltrials.gov/ct2/results?cond="familial+
adenomatous+polyposis"

Colon Cancer Alliance:
http://www.ccalliance.org

Colorectal Cancer Coalition:
http://fightcolorectalcancer.org

Global Genes:
http://globalgenes.org

Hereditary Colon Cancer Takes Guts:
http://www.hcctakesguts.org

Rare Science:
http://rarescience.org

ACKNOWLEDGEMENTS

There are many whose encouragement and patient tolerance of my first-time author anxieties helped pull *Summer's Complaint* from my head and heart to the pages you've just read. It is those individuals who exemplify (as Naomi Shihab Nye so eloquently reminds us) that "kindness is the deepest thing inside." Simple acknowledgement of their contributions throughout the writing of my family's story seems entirely inadequate, because my gratitude is so great.

To my friend Sarah Webber, who responded to my declaration that, "I think I should write a book about my family," with, "It's about damn time," and to my friend and colleague Monica Schultz who challenged me to show up for coffee with the first chapter in hand "...or else": I am forever grateful for your support and motivation.

To the Shryer Avenue kids and neighbors, Parkview Junior High classmates, and the wonderful people who came and went (and came and stayed) during my formative years: it has only been through all of you that this telling of my family's struggle has finally become possible. I was incredibly fortunate to grow up in "The Neighborhood" in Roseville, Minnesota and to know such wonderful people. You are far too numerous to name, but if you knew my parents or any one of their eight children, it's you I'm speaking of. Thank you.

To D.J. Schuette, my editor and publishing consultant at Critical Eye, who gently reminded me that adjectives are my friends and who talked me off the ledge multiple times when the self-doubt set in: you many never understand the depth of my gratitude for your advice and counsel. Many thanks.

To the great minds and students of science, medicine, social work, and psychology working on behalf of those with inherited cancer syndromes: I hope our story inspires and motivates you every day and reminds you of the great work you chose to pursue. Never give up that vital quest for knowledge. All humanity benefits from your endeavors. You are the future.

To those who not only diagnose and treat patients with genetic conditions, but who are also there to listen to the concerns and answer the endless questions of their families: your passion for medicine and the compassion for those under your care exemplifies the "heal" in healthcare.

To the people living with familial adenomatous polyposis and other inherited cancer syndromes: stay strong, always. I truly believe with all of the advancements being made every day that the random events that shape our lives will eventually be made "less random." We will be the beneficiaries of science and medical innovations that our parents and grandparents could only imagine.

To Paul Schultz, MD, my doctor of twenty-eight years and a family friend and confidante for over forty-five: there aren't words enough to express our appreciation. Thank you for giving us so many memories that we might never have had otherwise. You quite literally saved our lives.

To my Devils Lake kin: I'm so happy to have met you all in person. One of the greatest joys of pulling *Summer's Complaint* together was reconnecting with my mother's North Dakota roots.

To my husband, Bill, who encouraged me to write every day, even if it meant I spent way too much time sitting in the big grey chair by the fireplace, head down and typing furiously while surrounded by mountains of paper: You knew how important this book was to me. Thank you for your support and patience.

To my children, Alexander, Kelsey, and Adele, who constantly amaze and inspire me: my greatest achievement, my most profound blessing, is being your mom.

And to my siblings, nieces, and nephews, both those living and those who've already arrived on that distant horizon: despite everything we've been through, we did our best. Mom and Dad, Grandma "C," and Grandpa Jerry would be proud. This book is for us.

ABOUT THE AUTHOR

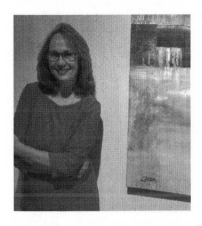

Laura Kieger has had a passion for writing since the first grade when she crayoned her debut short story about Penley, a pudgy penguin determined to fly. Her roles as an entrepreneur, parent, health advocate, and human resources professional in the medical field have all contributed to her desire to connect with others through the written word.

As a native Minnesotan and alumnus of the University of Minnesota, Laura is a huge Golden Gophers fan. She and her husband Bill raised their three kids, Alexander, Kelsey and Adele in the Twin Cities enjoying all the state has to offer—including it's character-building winters. *Summer's Complaint* is Laura's first book. Visit her website at www.laurakieger.com.

Front Cover Photo: Colleen Miller (Christensen), age one, with her parents, Reggie and Cecilia, circa 1931.

Made in the USA
Lexington, KY
23 February 2018